THE DNA GUIDE FOR ADOPTEES:

How to use genealogy and genetics to uncover your roots, connect with your biological family, and better understand your medical history.

By Brianne Kirkpatrick, MS, LCGC and Shannon Combs-Bennett, QG, PLCGS

CAMILLUS

The DNA Guide for Adoptees: How to use genealogy and genetics to uncover your roots, connect with your biological family, and better understand your medical history.

ISBN: 978-1-7337343-0-1

Library of Congress Control Number: 2019904219

Printed in the United States.

Cover design ©2019 by Charlotte's Web Creations

Author headshots ©2019 by Shutterbug's Creations

Table of Contents

Introduction

Welcome to *The DNA Guide for Adoptees: How to use genealogy and genetics to uncover your roots, connect with your biological family, and better understand your medical history.* If you are an adoptee, there is likely missing information about your past and you hope to change that. You have come to the right place!

People have different reasons for wanting to fill in the gaps in their history. You might be seeking a birth parent or sibling or hoping to connect with other biological family. Learning about your ethnic background might motivate you. Or, perhaps medical information matters most. For many adoptees, a combination of factors drives them to seek answers.

This book is for you if you hope that DNA testing might open up the search for information about yourself, your origins, and your future. We worked hard to compile the resources in this book and explain in plain English how DNA and genealogical records fit together like the pieces of a puzzle. In the chapters that follow, you will come face-to-face with questions about health, ancestry, biological family, and DNA.

Why DNA testing, and why now?

DNA testing is a game-changer for people researching family connections. Many recent advances have made it possible for adoptees to search for answers more easily than they could have done even a few years ago. Consider the following changes:

- At-home DNA tests have grown in number and dropped in price.

- Millions of people use software to build and track their family trees and share results online.

- Billions of vital records, legal files, and other documents are available online.

- Social networks and search engines make it easy to find and connect to people all over the world.

- Adoptees are sharing their DNA stories publicly, through television shows and other media.

While advances in DNA testing are exciting and useful, there are real limitations. We will be the first to acknowledge that DNA does not hold all of the answers for everyone, but it plays an important role for many adoptees hoping to learn more about themselves and their genetics. In some cases, DNA testing has helped adoptees discover unknown medical risks, which is invaluable in situations where little or no family health history is available.

You may have already started down the path of DNA testing, or it may be entirely new to you. No matter where you are starting, we have worked to make the information in this book interesting, useful, and easy to understand. We include real-life examples, fictionalized scenarios, and advice gathered from adoptees to make this book relevant no matter your prior experience with DNA.

Why this book?

As two women active in the genetic genealogy community, our decision to work together on *The DNA Guide for Adoptees* came from a desire to provide a comprehensive resource about DNA testing that pulls everything into one place. What you learn from testing your DNA can have a profound impact on you, your family members, and even future generations.

Information can be a powerful thing. As mothers, daughters, sisters, spouses, and friends, we have seen how the discovery of new information can impact relationships. As writers and professionals with unique and diverse experiences in genetics, genealogy, and counseling support, we also know the journey through DNA and a search for family can be emotional for many people. We have worked professionally and personally with adoptees, and we understand some of the unique challenges you face.

This book will provide you with practical advice on topics such as medical and genealogical DNA testing, handling emotional aspects of the search, and recommended resources to help take your research efforts to the next level. What helps one person may not be relevant for others, so we cover different approaches suitable for different situations.

The book is broken down into four main sections:

- **Part 1: Getting started.** This covers first steps, learning the options open to you and your rights, and emotional preparation. (Chapters 1-12)

- **Part 2: Bringing science and research together through genetic genealogy.** This section introduces genetics and the finer details of genealogical DNA testing. (Chapters 13-17)

- **Part 3: What to do after DNA testing is done.** Here you will find guidance and tips for managing and organizing the information you discover along the way and suggested wording for reaching out to newly-discovered DNA relatives. (Chapters 18-21)

- **Part 4: Health and DNA.** This special section covers medical genetic testing with the unique needs of adoptees in mind. A bonus chapter addressing issues for adoptive parents and minor children is also included. (Chapters 22-28)

To you, our readers, we wish you the best in your search for information. A book cannot complete the journey for you, but we hope it will serve as a source of encouragement to get started, a guide to practical resources to use in your search, and a place to return for continued support.

Brianne Kirkpatrick, MS, LCGC
Shannon Combs-Bennett, QG, PLCGS

Part 1: Getting Started

Being a part of the online community of people doing genealogy and DNA work related to adoption, it has become a daily norm to see posts such as these:

> *"Found my birth mom today! Reaching out now …"*

> *"I finally did it! Found my birth family and know their names, after 45 years."*

> *"My original birth certificate arrived, and I finally have learned the name I was given at birth by my biological mom."*

> *"Figured out another adoption mystery for someone today, and in record time!"*

There are many stories like these, often condensed into just a sentence or two. These shortened tales of discovery obscure the blood, sweat, and tears that people went through to uncover the identities of their birth families. Just the thought of getting started on a search might be overwhelming, especially if you have already attempted to search for information in the past without success.

Recently, an email arrived in Brianne's inbox. It was from an adult adoptee named Judey. In the email, Judey outlined the story of her search for birth family. It had taken decades, cost thousands of dollars in fees to researchers and a personal investigator, and resulted in one disappointment after another. She eventually gave up her search and pushed the thoughts aside for twenty years.

In a twist of events that could be a novel, Judey and her birth mother Ginna each decided to take a DNA test, mainly for ethnicity reasons. Because children receive half of their DNA from a parent, the DNA testing service was able to match them as parent/child. They connected as a result of DNA, an outcome that paper records could not enable. Judey reached out to Brianne to tell her story, wanting it to be shared with others as a message of hope to other adoptees not to give up their search.

Not all adoption-related searches turn out the same as Judey's, and not all reunions happen because of a parent and child independently taking DNA tests. Documents, like an original birth certificate and adoption paperwork, are often enough to allow someone to identify and connect with a biological relative. When DNA is involved, the test often connects an adoptee to distant family rather than close. The adoptee must then do some detective work to figure out how the people they match from DNA testing are related to a birth parent.

It may seem that there are only two possible outcomes when you search for biological family: you either find family or do not. And, if your search is successful and you decide to reach out to biological relatives, there are two further possibilities: acceptance or rejection. In reality, there are countless outcomes to the search for information, and an indefinite number of possible endings to your story.

These first few chapters of *The DNA Guide for Adoptees* aim to prepare you to search for more information, no matter what the future might hold. Whether your goal is to have a reunion or only to determine your biological origins, the next few chapters offer details on places to seek out information. We pose questions that can guide your search and prepare you for various outcomes.

Chapter 1:
Getting started on a search

The first step in any journey is the hardest one to take. But once you commit yourself and put the first foot in front of you, the steps that follow will be easier. Of course, there will be bumps, dips, and detours along the way. But these are a part of most life journeys, so expect them when setting out to connect with other people and your own past.

When searching for answers related to adoption that require digging into documents or your DNA, it is important to identify the motivating factors for your search. Knowing the underlying reasons will help determine the path ahead. These might be the types of questions to ask yourself:

- Do I seek a better understanding of the circumstances around my adoption?

- Is it possible to locate (and build relationships with) relatives from my biological family?

- Is my primary goal to gather medical information, to better understand my health or that of my children?

- Do I have one burning question or many?

- How will I know if I have found my answer or finished my search?

This last question is perhaps the most important. It is worth putting some thought toward a specific goal or set of desired outcomes, with the understanding that the search might be fast and easy, or it might be long and arduous. For some people, no matter the outcome, the search for the truth is worth it, even if all the questions cannot be fully answered.

Not everyone desires a reunion or relationship with birth family members. Some adoptees simply want to know their biological origins and who their birth parents are. Do not feel the need to equate identification of your family with a reunion if it is not right for you.

Some people are private and do not have any desire for a reunion or any situation that would lead to an outward display of emotions. No matter your personal feelings about all of these factors, they are valid.

Keep your goal in mind as you progress through the book and pay attention to where your imagination goes. Let your instincts tell you when you need to keep searching and when it is time to rest. You may be able to do everything on your own or may reach a point at which you need to call in back-up support.

Who to tell, and when to start?

Some people hesitate to tell others about a search for birth family, perhaps because of worry about a negative reaction or causing hurt to loved ones. Others are willing to confide in family members or long-time friends who will support them along the way.

An adoption-related search can create a ripple effect that touches others. Whether you are the person who was adopted, a birth parent, or a member of the adoptive family, a search can bring up latent feelings and memories. Bringing them up to the surface can have an impact on your life and for others as well, emotionally and in other ways. Siblings—both birth and adoptive—can also be affected. So can spouses, significant others, children, friends, and even coworkers.

Marie, an adoptee, was in her mid-50s and her adoptive parents in their mid-80s when she began to actively search for biological relatives. A few decades earlier, Marie had brought up the topic of her adoption with her mother, but quickly dropped it when her mother grew upset. Her mother ended the conversation abruptly by declaring, "You are our daughter, and that is that."

As she got older, Marie realized time was running out to find out details about any medical conditions that run in her biological family. She also realized she might miss out on the only chance to meet her biological parents before they died. She decided to begin searching, but only told her husband, adult children, and best friend.

You may be a person who finds it easier to be open with everyone and feel no qualms about the reaction of others. Maybe you are reluctant like Marie was for many years. Whatever your reasons, know that it is okay whether you share your intentions openly or only with a close circle. Only you know what feels right.

Complete these sentences (in your head or on paper) as you think about starting or resuming your search:

- One thing holding me back is ...
- I will know the time is right to search when ...
- My biggest fear about searching is ...
- I get excited or anxious when I think about ...

Who you tell and when you tell them depends a lot on your unique circumstances and relationships. You might start by identifying the people you have turned to for support and encouragement in the past and reflect on how you will cope with any conflict and frustration you may confront.

Navigating family dynamics

There is no "right" time in life to start a search for biological family; it is a personal choice for everyone. You might have reached a life milestone such as turning 18 or starting a family. Perhaps you or your child has developed a medical condition, and the timing of your search has become urgent for that reason. You might have waited until after the death of your adoptive parents, as many people in this situation describe feeling free to undertake a search in a way they did not before.

Even if someone in your life has explicitly asked you not to search, you may still opt to move forward. Think through how you might best explain to them your reasons for deciding to search, and how you will handle sharing information about what you discover.

Sometimes searching leads people to new relationships that can disrupt family dynamics and friendships, either temporarily or for a long time. This is normal. Change can be painful for different people for different reasons.

The search experience and the impact on day-to-day life differ for each person. In addition, your feelings can fluctuate over time. Strong emotions, whether they are generally positive or negative, can impact your ability to carry on as usual at home, school, or work.

Whether through spoken or written word, communicate as clearly and openly as you can with those around you. Encourage everyone to look for support, and do this yourself as well. We will dig a little deeper into this topic and mention sources of emotional support later on.

Coping with painful experiences along the way

For many people, the search for biological family is exciting and leads to a happy or satisfying outcome for them. But what about those whose search is hard and leads to painful experiences? If you have imagined what it might be like to search for family, and if you have imagined a warm and emotional reunion with them, it can be disappointing if reality does not pan out that way.

As uncomfortable as is it to think about a negative outcome, the truth is some adoptees experience what is referred to by some as secondary rejection by birth family. One or more birth family members may deny they are related to you, or they may refuse any contact. Some adoptees have had hateful and hurtful things said to them. Communication may begin and then suddenly stop without an explanation.

These behaviors may be temporary. The reactions of birth relatives sometimes happen because some people need more time to adjust with the change in their family or someone does not know how to proceed when a family secret has been brought to light.

Sometimes the difficulty or refusal to communicate goes in the other direction as well, with an adoptee not wishing to reunite with a searching biological parent or other family member who wants to connect with them.

In Brianne's family's experience, for example, Brianne's grandmother was raised by kin after the death of her mother and abandonment by her father as a young girl. When her father attempted to re-enter his daughter's life in adulthood, it was unwelcomed. The father and daughter did not reconnect before his death, but other relatives in the family have reunited many decades later, aided by genealogical searching and DNA testing.

Later in this part of the book, we cover the different types of support. The resources section at the end also contains links to podcasts, support groups, and websites created for searching adoptees that can help if you struggle emotionally.

Chapter 2:
Understanding records related to adoptions

Many adoptees assume the search for biological family will begin online or with a DNA test. For some people, a more effective starting point may be official documents and genealogical records. We explore this type of information next to help you figure out which direction you might start looking first.

Rights to access identifying versus non-identifying information

The types of information contained in adoption records can be classified as either **identifying** (ID) or **non-identifying** (non-ID). The difference between them is whether the information might be able to identify a specific person or people, or if it is general enough that the information could describe many people.

Non-identifying information (or "non-ID") in records may include the date and place of an adopted child's birth, age and physical description of birth parents, medical history reported by the birth parents, reasons provided for the child's placement for adoption, and the existence of other children born to each parent.

Identifying information will contain additional details the agency has on file about the birth parents and the adoption. It may include the real name of a birth mother, and if reported, the birth father. There may be details into the circumstances surrounding the adoption. In some cases there could be a current or most recently known address listed for a birth parent.

There are state-by-state rules that govern rights to information and who can access which type of information. Knowing your legal rights to ID and non-ID information about your birth and adoption is an excellent foundation on which to begin a search. You can save time by learning what information you are already entitled to. The number of states and countries granting adoptees more access to their information is growing.

Connect with adoption registries (see Chapter 3) that exist in the state or country where you were adopted, and determine which state department(s) holds record of the information you are seeking. You may learn everything you need to identify and locate biological family simply by requesting documents from the office, agency, or department that possesses them.

State-by-state differences

The Adoptee Rights Law website, adopteerightslaw.com, is a source for information on legal rights to documents relating to United States adoptions. Rights and access are continually changing, usually for the better, as adoption rights advocates lobby for access to records and adoptee-friendly legislation in different states. Note that each state differs in what records can be accessed by an adoptee searching for birth parents.

An excellent all-in-one resource for learning about what laws affect you if you were adopted in United States is the Child Welfare Information Gateway run by the U.S. Department of Health and Human Services. This resource is invaluable for understanding what the current laws are in each state. Another helpful resource is the American Adoption Congress. Its website, americanadoptioncongress.org, also maintains current information on which states restrict access to records.

As an example of how rights differ from one state to another, consider New Hampshire and Vermont. At the time of writing, New Hampshire is one of the states that allows adult adoptees to have unrestricted access to their original birth certificate. Right across the state line in Vermont, however, an adoptee needs a court order or must have already received identifying information from the state's adoption registry before they are granted access to their original birth certificate.

> **Insider Tip:** To get a complete look at what adoption-related documents you may have access to, there is an excellent brochure by the Child Welfare Information Gateway, U.S. Department of Health and Human Services (DHHS). Their website is kept up to date on the laws of each state. You can download a PDF copy from their website or get a print copy at a DHHS office.

Rules surrounding your legal rights to access records can have caveats, and accessing ID and non-ID information is not straightforward. Indiana is one of the states that recently changed the law, granting adult adoptees access to an original birth certificate and other information about their adoption. However, birth parents have rights to limit what information about themselves is available to others. Here is an example of the steps required in Indiana:

Steps to obtaining information from the Indiana State Department of Health Mutual Consent Registry:

1. Fill out form 47896 for identifying information (available online at forms.in.gov).

2. Fill out form 47897 for non-identifying information (available online at forms.in.gov).

3. Copy or photograph your driver's license or state-issued photo ID and include it with the forms.

4. Submit forms and copy of your ID by mail to the address on the bottom of the form OR submit forms online to the email address provided.

Indiana's law, like some other states, is complicated in that it permits release of the original birth certificate to an adoptee, but with certain restrictions. If a birth parent requests an intermediary be involved, for example, the permission for the original birth certificate is revoked. Some people call this a "mother, may I" provision and rightly argue that states like Indiana are not fully granting adoptees their rights.

Other states will have similar processes in place to make sure that documents are released to those who have a legal right to them. Rules may differ if you were born in one state and your adoption took place in another. You may have to set aside some time to understand the nuances of the laws in the state or states where you were born and adopted.

> **Insider Tip:** It is not just an adoptee who can access his or her original birth certificate. Some states allow the over-21 adult adoptee, adoptive parent, birth parent, birth sibling, spouse, or other relative of a deceased adoptee or birth parent to request a copy.

Records search for international adoptions

There are some special issues to be aware of if you were born outside of the U.S.

The ability to search for and find records differs for those adopted across national borders. Many agencies that handle international adoptions offer post-adoption services that may include counseling and will provide adoption records when requested.

Some adoptees have been surprised to discover not everything was done legally, or that proper papers to finalize citizenship were not completed upon their arrival in the U.S. as foreign-born adopted children. Legislation called the Child Citizenship Act of 2000 has provided citizenship assurance for many adoptees, but there are tens of thousands of adoptees in the U.S. who were born internationally, are not legal citizens, and are not protected by the act.

Adoptee Rights Campaign is an advocacy group for intercountry adoptees. You may wish to connect with the group or locate an attorney to speak with as you begin to search for records related to your international/intercountry adoption. This is important if you are concerned about your citizenship paperwork or learn more about common yet ethically and legally questionable practices occurring around the time of your birth and adoption.

Consumer DNA testing (covered in Part 2) can bypass the search for biological relatives based on documentation. Success with this path for international adoptees depends on whether DNA testing is available to consumers and widely done where they were born.

As the databases grow larger, the possibility of matching with distant cousins and more closely related biological family also grows. Because the use of DNA tests is expanding worldwide, the chances are improving for international adoptees to make progress in their family searches. We briefly cover another search option for international adoptees – that of mutual consent registries – in the next chapter.

Chapter 3:
People and places to go
for information

Information about births and adoptions are often spread out, with a birth certificate on file in one state department and an adoption file held by another. There are people and systems set up to help you gain access, but navigating the system is not always easy. Confidential intermediaries, registries, and DNA testing fit into many current searches.

Confidential intermediary

A **confidential intermediary** (**CI**) is a person who can be involved in managing the release of information and communication between an adoptee and birth relatives. CIs are individuals who have access to the records. Many have gone through a training program to become certified and are court-appointed. They serve a role in tracking down and communicating with both parties and release to each party what is permitted by law and approved by those who are contacted.

There are requirements that must be met before using the services of a CI, and these vary by state. Not all states employ CIs. In those that do, they may require you to be age 21 or require that your adoption must have taken place during a particular time frame (between 1945 and 1980, for example).

States that do not use CIs sometimes have an affidavit system through which birth family members can either file their consent to release ID information or register a refusal to be contacted. This is sometimes called a consent, waiver, or authorization form. An Internet search can help you locate CI services or an affidavit system in your state of adoption, if they exist.

Registries

A **registry** is a set of information (usually name and contact information) used for any different number of reasons. You may be able to find out if someone is already searching for you by looking into existing adoption registries. Online registries specifically set up for adoption-related searches are typically free of charge. Also called mutual consent registries, these sites maintain contact information and details for people who are looking for a biological relative and want to be found. Both parties are notified by a third party if they both join the same registry and are interested in contact.

Registries are not a guaranteed way to reconnect with a biological relative, since not every adoptee, birth parent, or birth relative knows about the registries. Nevertheless, they have resulted in successful reunions countless times.

You can maximize your chances of a registry connecting you to biological family by finding and signing up for as many relevant registries (often based on where your adoption took place) as you can.

> **Insider Tip:** Some of the more well-known registries include Adopted.com, Adoption Reunion Registry, ALMA Society, and International Soundex Reunion Registry. Additional registries can be found by doing an Internet search or by asking support groups and online groups where members are familiar with the options where your adoption took place.

There are differences from state to state about who may use adoption registry and CI services and whether approval by the court is required. In Illinois, for example, an adult adoptee, their birth parents, and adoptive parents may file a petition to use CI services without a court order. Birth siblings of an adoptee are also permitted to use CI services but require permission of the court.

If the access to records is restricted where your birth and adoption took place, or your work with a CI does not lead to answers, do not settle. Some people hire an attorney or a private investigator and succeed in gaining access to records that way.

DNA testing

DNA testing provides a compelling alternative to the middlemen, bureaucrats, and other adoption gatekeepers who once controlled information about adoptees and birth families. DNA has also changed how, when, and with whom adoptees first connect to biological family. As you might expect from the title of this book, we cover this topic in great detail in later sections.

Starting in the early 2000s, online DNA testing services were first used by genealogists researching family origins. Because of how well it worked, use quickly spread to people trying to connect with biological family.

DNA might not automatically connect you with a birth parent or sibling. A more typical scenario is to discover you match a long list of distant cousins, which you then need to research and communicate with. On the other hand, you may discover someone who is a close match, and your search for biological family wraps up quickly.

Some regions of the world still have low rates of DNA testing, meaning any family matches may be distant and not helpful to the search. As databases grow larger and more diverse, the usefulness of DNA testing will grow for many.

Insider Tip: If you choose to go the DNA testing route, learn about your rights. Submitting a DNA sample to a for-profit company or research project also involves giving up some aspects of your rights, ownership of your DNA information, and control over how your data is stored, sold, and shared with others. Once permission is granted, you may not be able to resume full control. This is not only true of DNA data, but also any other type of information you submit, including names, age, relationships, and family trees. Read the Terms of Service and Privacy Policy to know what you are agreeing to. These documents contain details about what the company will do with your DNA sample after they run your test and with whom they will share your information. The fine print lays out what is in your control and what you can do if you change your mind and wish to remove your data in the future. Understand that the terms can and do change with time, sometimes without warning and sometimes after a company has already violated the terms of the agreement.

Since the introduction of DNA testing, family other than an adoptee and their birth parent participate in adoption-related family searches. Intentional searching for (and unintentional discoveries of) biological family now often includes biological siblings, cousins, aunts, uncles, and even grandparents.

Sometimes DNA testing identifies a sibling or close cousin of a birth parent first, even before the mother or father is ever identified. Relatives who never knew a baby or child was placed for adoption are suddenly privy to a family secret, and they must decide how to proceed. This change in the way some adopted family members are discovered requires balancing the needs of more people in a family than ever before.

This involvement of more family has marked a major shift, removing a level of privacy once assumed for those most closely involved in adoptions. It has shifted the discovery of adoption-related information into the hands of the individuals who have decided to order a DNA test.

How relatives react to being contacted out of the blue varies from family to family and even within families. There is no guidebook for how to navigate the waters of DNA testing, but we are beginning to learn from the stories of others who have done it.

The combination approach

You might make the best progress by using a combination of DNA testing and requesting records and documents. The best way to determine which approach will be best for you is to connect with an adoptee support group or organization from the state or country of your birth. Those who have undertaken a search before will know which DNA tests are most likely to be helpful and where you will find the right forms to submit to request your records.

Some adoptees will choose to involve a professional counselor or professional searcher to support them through a search, whether using records, DNA testing, or both. The next section covers the topic of identifying potential sources of help to turn to, which may be important whether your approach involves DNA or a different search method.

Chapter 4: Finding support

Other people who can help with a search

There are other types of helpers and professionals who work with adoptees and birth family to help them make progress in their search. Some are paid for their time and expertise, while others volunteer their services.

Many have highly-developed research skills for locating genealogy and adoption records. These specialized skills allow them to quickly navigate publicly available information, historical databases, and in some cases, DNA results.

A **search angel** is an experienced researcher who volunteers their time to individual cases. They enjoy working with adoptees, typically because they have been through a search for biological family themselves or on behalf of someone they know, and they want to share their skills to help others. Many search angels know the ins and outs of searching for information in specific states or countries. They also have personalities that help form bonds of trust and empathy as they guide others through the search process.

Genetic genealogists have become adept at using DNA information to piece together how individuals and their families are connected. Many are self-taught and do not have a formal scientific education. They may use information from DNA testing combined with genealogical research to construct a person's possible family tree. Often these trees begin with a deceased ancestor and are built down to current-day, living family members. Those who do this work full-time often refer to themselves as professional genetic genealogists.

Since genetic genealogists working professionally and volunteers acting as search angels do not have a process for becoming degreed and certified, there is potential for more variability in the type of support, information, and services each can provide. You may reach a point in your search where you reach a dead end; locating one of these helpers may allow you to continue moving forward in your search.

> **Insider Tip:** If you are unable to find someone who can help you on a volunteer basis, or if your volunteer hits a wall in their research, hiring assistance from a professional genetic genealogist may be invaluable. It may save both time and frustration to work with a paid professional, even if only temporarily. Word-of-mouth from others who have benefitted from the help of an experienced search angel or a genetic genealogist might point you toward the person or people who can offer guidance and assistance.

There is growing support for adoptees who decide to search for more information about their origins. In addition to friends and family members, adoptees can connect with professional counselors, experienced searchers, and other adoptees who understand the emotional and practical challenges adoptees face when seeking to connect with biological family.

> **Insider Tip:** Outside support can make a world of difference. Online communities, like the Facebook groups *DNA Detectives*, *Adoption Search & Reunion* , and *Search Squad*, are large groups dedicated to helping people make connections to biological family. There are additional smaller groups that aim to provide emotional support to various people involved in a family search or reunion. In some areas, there are in-person support groups and small group therapy sessions for adoptees that meet on a regular basis.

Locating a therapist or counselor

Working one-on-one with a trained counselor or therapist before, during, or after the search has been helpful to many people. These professionals can be a source of support for times when you are going through a major life change. Some people have ongoing relationships with their counselors, while others may only visit a few times.

There are various types of counselors and therapists, each with different training and professional skill sets. Note that all licensed professionals working in the mental health field are expected to recognize their limits. It is common for these professionals to refer a client to a different type of professional when the needs for support go beyond the professional's training and expertise.

One adoptee in her 40s who we spoke with told us that she had benefitted from working with a therapist specially trained in working with adoptees. She worked with the therapist before starting her search, describing the therapy as a process of resolving the trauma and grief that arose from being separated from biological family. Because of how helpful she found it to be, she always advises other adoptees to consider doing the same, *before* starting with DNA testing or different types of searching.

Some people refer to counselors with specialized knowledge or training as being *adoption competent*. These counselors are familiar with issues that can come into play during a search for biological family or as a result of a reunion. You might seek the support of an adoption competent counselor for any number of reasons, but particularly if you experience:

- The resurfacing of past trauma triggered by the search or reunion

- **Genetic sexual attraction** (GSA) with a biological relative (see Chapter 12)

- Discovery of upsetting circumstances around your adoption, such as conception from rape or incest (see Chapter 12)

> **Insider Tip:** Adoption competent therapists are prepared to recognize, understand, and address the common social and psychological challenges that arise in adoption situations. You can search for an adoption-competent therapist by researching online and by asking others in your geographical area or in the adoptee community. Some counselors work with clients remotely and others see clients only in person.

Chapter 5: Anxiety, fear, and expectation

Reece was a 20-something American college student adopted from Russia as an infant. She had been reluctant to get started on the search for birth family because she feared there would be no information available for her to uncover beyond what her parents received at the time of her adoption. She was also skeptical of DNA databases whose members were primarily American-born people.

In other words, the fear of finding nothing held Reece back. Fear and anxiety can be as big of a roadblock to you moving forward on a search as closed adoption records might be. Learning about anxiety and how to work with it can be key to your progress in your search. Read on if Reece's story resonates with you.

Anxiety triggers

There are all kinds of anxiety triggers associated with starting a search for biological family. Not knowing where to start can paralyze some people for years. The wait for documents or DNA test results can also be nerve-racking. When a piece of mail with an original birth certificate finally arrives, or an email pops up notifying you of new DNA results, you might notice your heart skip a beat as you wonder what you are about to learn.

Anxiety often boils down to a feeling of not being control. You may be terrified of uncovering something unexpected and upsetting, while at the same time be fearful that you will not discover anything at all. An overwhelming fear of rejection by birth family has been described by adoptees and holds many back.

These are all very real emotional experiences. It may help you to realize you are not alone or different for feeling the way you do and to realize that intense emotional reactions are normal.

Identifying your fears

Identifying and naming your fears can help you manage the anxiety you feel related to searching. This short exercise can help you get started. Complete the following sentences:

- I worry that ...
- I will be so upset if ...
- I am nervous to ...
- I will probably feel angry if...

Peeling back the layers of emotions and learning to identify them can be difficult if you were not brought up in a household that talked about emotions and feelings. Consider spending some time preparing yourself for the emotional journey and reach out to a counselor, friend, spouse, or another close confidant if you found it difficult to identify and name your worries and other emotions.

Insider Tip: There are many books written by adoptees that address the deeply emotional and traumatic aspects of adoption many people find it more difficult to talk about. Two to consider reading are Anne Heffron's *You Don't Look Adopted* or Nancy Newton Verrier's *The Primal Wound*.

Setting and managing expectations

Setting expectations at the start of a search can be challenging. There are so many unknowns, ranging from the time it takes to receive a requested birth certificate to the likelihood of getting a close family member match from DNA testing.

Some members of Facebook groups for adoption search support have posted about their disappointments. Finding no close matches after joining a DNA matching database can feel like rejection. "Why isn't my birth family already out there trying to find me?" has been a sentiment expressed by more than one person in these search groups who failed to have any close family member matches.

Even if you approach the search with a low bar, you might find your expectations dashed anyway. A search can take longer than expected, you might find a lack of close matches, or you might encounter people who refuse to respond to messages or close the door in your face.

It can be absolutely devastating when someone who has been searching for months or years finally finds a biological relative, and that person refuses contact. Or, the adoptee identifies a birth parent, but he or she has already died.

Not every story ends in heartbreak. Many searches for biological relatives have had positive outcomes. Every day it seems another story about a successful search pops up. Reunion videos are regularly posted on social networking sites, and some even make it into the popular media.

These stories are uplifting and provide hope. They show that for some adoptees, the search for biological family can lead to connecting with new relatives eager to meet and get to know them. These powerful stories often include elements of struggle and joy, and they give hope to others embarking on similar journeys.

As the public grows more and more aware of these types of reunions, there seems to be an increasing willingness to help with the search. Some people with DNA accounts have added the term "adoption friendly" or "DD" (for DNA detective) to their online profiles to let others know they are willing to communicate and help.

With every positive story shared on social media or reported by the media, the odds increase that you may discover a helper eager to assist you. You might even find a biological relative excited to help you trace the line to your birth parent(s).

Know that it is okay to have expectations. Your own story will have its unique twists, turns, struggles, and joys. It probably will not make it onto television or become a viral video, but that by no means minimizes its significance in the world or to your life.

Patience is a crucial virtue, as searching can be time-intensive. It may take weeks for a state agency to respond to a request for a vital record. Participating in DNA testing requires ordering a test kit, preparing the spit or swab sample, shipping it, and waiting for the results. The process can take months to complete – and it may take years before a close match appears.

Some steps will be in your control and on your time. Some will not. Be persistent in your search, but also patient when things slow down. Realize the journey does not end when you find the person or people you are looking for, as one adoptee told us. Finding your birth relatives may be the first step in a life-long journey of getting to know them and to find out answers to long-standing questions.

Dealing with frustration during the search

Marilyn was an adoptee who posted to an online Facebook group about her frustrations with her search. She had spent hundreds of hours scouring the family trees of her DNA matches and following recommended steps she had learned about using the information to puzzle out her biological mother and father. She ran into one dead end after another.

"What a waste!" she posted to the online forum. "I should have used all that time researching to learn a new language instead!"

Another adoptee, Lynne, gave advice from her personal experience. "When you're looking for blood relatives, it's easy to get discouraged," she explained to Shannon. "When you're at that point, take a break from the search effort and do something fun. Give your brain a break!"

> **Insider Tip:** You might reach a point of extreme aggravation, especially if your search is going slowly. At times, you might feel like giving up. If this happens, do not lose hope. Taking a break is okay. Pick up the search again when you feel refreshed. Genealogists are introducing new tools and techniques for analyzing DNA matches, and one of these new tools might be the key in making progress.

It is helpful to recognize that media portrayals of successful adoptee searches and reunions do not paint the whole picture. Television shows tend to skip over the challenges that arose during a search. The shows also fail to capture the hundreds of hours of self-directed learning, educational training, and practice the experienced searchers already had under their belts.

The challenges faced by brand new searchers (sometimes called "newbies") and people who encounter dead ends or disappointing outcomes in a family search are seldom chosen to have their stories featured by the media. Add to this sunny advertising by the major DNA companies, and it is no wonder many people are disillusioned by a challenging search.

These short highlights in the media of DNA family discoveries stop before the next chapter of the story. In the months and years that follow an adoptee's identification of biological family, in-person meetings sometimes happen or do not. New relationships may begin to develop, or might not.

Many adoptees have described that finding family has been positive experience but also the start of new bumps in the road. If you expect to find new family members, expect to put in time and effort to develop new relationships as well.

Chapter 6:
Common ancestors and living relatives

A DNA test is not a magic wand that instantly rolls out your entire family tree when results come back. You may be one of the lucky ones whose DNA test immediately returns a match to a close family member, making your search short. Many others find that they only match to distant family like second or third cousins, then they must figure out how they connect to them.

Sometimes you must turn into an online detective and track down living people to figure out who are the members of your biological family. This chapter introduces the skills you must develop to be able to make use of DNA tests (explained in Part 2) and family trees in your search for other people related to you.

Relying on other peoples' family trees

It is quite common to turn to other people's family trees. The trees of your DNA test matches that are posted online are one of the best places to start. Millions of people have conducted genealogical research to learn about their own roots and posted the results online. When you match someone by DNA, it may be possible to figure out where you fit on their trees by putting together what you know about the location of your birth and adoption and how that fits with people in their tree.

There are challenges to relying on other people's family tree research. But at the same time, if you use DNA to search for family, it is vital. Here are some challenges you might face:

- Not everyone is precise or consistent when they build their family trees.

- Unknown family secrets can hide actual genetic relationships and might mislead you.
- Very few family trees posted online are large, detailed, accurate, and error-free.
- Your parent also might be adopted (or have misattributed parentage) and thus might not show up in the family trees you review.
- When you reach out to communicate with a promising match, they may not respond.
- People who do respond might not have helpful information.
- Someone who responds initially may quit communicating with you later.

Using DNA results and searching family trees is a bit like sorting out the pieces of a jigsaw puzzle. You may run into challenges if you have to rely on the family research of others. But with documents, DNA testing, and some of the tools discussed in later chapters, it is possible to use DNA results and family trees to track down relatives. The stories of success you read in online groups and hear about in the media have relied on these techniques and demonstrate that they work!

People-searching sites

Where the names and other detailed information in family trees stop is where the living family members start. Online trees do not list the names of people marked as "living," so that is where you will need to pick up the search yourself. Searching for living people is harder, but it can be done.

Obituaries are often the most useful source of information because they are a place where a deceased person is listed along with the names of their living family (spouse, siblings, children, and grandchildren, for example).

The following chart lists the various websites where you can often search for the identity and contact information for living people.

Been Verified (beenverified.com)	Find A Grave (findagrave.com)
Classmates (classmates.com)	Genealogy Bank (genealogybank.com)
David Gray's People Finder (davidgraypeoplefinder.com)	Geni (geni.com)
DNA.Land (dna.land)	Google (google.com)
DOB search (dobsearch.com)	LinkedIn (linkedin.com)
Facebook (facebook.com)	Newspapers (newspapers.com)
Family Search (familysearch.org)	Pipl (pipl.com)
Family Tree Now (familytreenow.com)	Public Data (publicdata.com)

Chapter 7:
Learning from others

Sometimes barriers you face are that people you expect will have information are either unwilling or unable to give it. Pregnancy conception as a result of a one-time encounter means the mother may not know the identity of the birth father. If someone has already died, you might not have the opportunity to get all of your questions answered.

The experiences that others have been through can help you overcome the challenges and barriers you may run into as you make progress in your search. Consider the situations of these three adoptees: Alice, Laura, and June.

Alice's story

Alice was conceived as the result of a one-night stand and was relinquished at birth by her birth mother. Alice found her birth mother using non-ID information from her adoption file and the assistance of a confidential intermediary. Because her biological father was unknown to her birth mother, Alice turned to DNA. The closest DNA matches Alice found all led straight back to her birth mother's family. Did this mean her biological mother and father were related? Or did it simply indicate her biological father's side had not tested yet?

The anxiety from not knowing and not being able to get straight answers made things difficult for Alice. Many months later, she was still unable to solve the mystery, and the anxiety continued to plague her daily. After hearing about a free analysis tool available online called "Are your parents related?" (see Chapter 21), Alice decided she was ready to explore this possibility using her DNA results. She was comforted when the result stated that based on the markers analyzed from her DNA raw data file, it was unlikely her parents were related within recent generations.

Eventually, a search angel helped Alice try a new approach with her DNA match results where they grouped her matches together based on who matched each other and then color-coded them. This allowed them to put aside matches that were maternal relatives and to narrow down the search to a particular branch where it appeared all of her paternal-side relatives were matching. The search angel scoured the family trees of people in that colored grouping, and it led her to two brothers on the family tree who were potentially the birth father. Either brother could have been the father based on his age and location at the time of Alice's conception.

Using the two brothers' names, they searched Facebook and YouTube and were able to locate information, including one video. Alice's birth mother recognized the name and the face of the man in the video and was able to confirm he likely was Alice's birth father. DNA testing, family trees, and Internet research had led them to the likely birth father of Alice, and if he (or one of his children) were to DNA test, Alice and her search angel could be absolutely sure they had found the right person. Alice currently is thinking about how to reach out to her potential birth father who as of right now has no idea she exists.

Laura's story

After the death of her mother, Laura overheard a rumor that she had been adopted at birth. Her father confirmed the rumor was true. Laura sought out an online support group for late-discovery adoptees like herself and decided to take a DNA test. The test led her to a half-brother and a second cousin. Laura began to communicate with these DNA matches and determined from information she had such as location and age that the half-brother was likely through her birth father and the second cousin through her birth mother. They were able to drill down into each family to determine the likely identities of the birth parents and where their lives had intersected. Testing other family members helped confirm the theory.

Unfortunately, Laura's birth mother had died young (age 42) from breast cancer, so Laura never had a chance to meet her. Her birth father also had died before Laura had a chance to meet him. Laura was disappointed that she was never able to meet them and ask them about the circumstances of her birth and adoption. The DNA testing ultimately brought her in touch with half-siblings on both sides of her birth family, and they were welcoming of her. Laura has met them in person, and she enjoys visiting and traveling around the country to visit with them when the time allows.

June's story

June was adopted at birth in 1931 in Virginia which is a state that has sealed records. She had already tried testing at two DNA companies, 23andMe and MyHeritage, in her search without receiving a close match. When she spoke with Brianne about her birth family search, Brianne recommended trying AncestryDNA test next. The results came back with four matches estimated at the level of first cousins. Because two of these matches had family trees built and open for public viewing, Brianne was able to research the matches and identify June's biological mother and father in less than four hours.

June and Brianne discussed how to reach out to the DNA matches and came up with a plan. Their messages were met with confusion at first, since no living family members were aware June had been born and adopted out of the family. But to everyone's pleasure, members from both sides of the family began to communicate, welcomed June, and sent her pictures.

After 88 years of not knowing the family she was born to or where her personal traits came from, June was able to see she shared red hair with biological family and that her musical and artistic talents appeared to be family traits as well. June always said she felt she was connected to family of many different types and was loved and cared for by many, but the connection to biological family brought her a kind of joy and satisfaction she had not been able to experience before.

These three stories highlight different experiences, challenges, and outcomes for adoptees who turned to DNA to identify their biological origins. While there is no singular adoptee experience, there are many shared experiences. Others have been through and learned the ways to search for biological family, and many of them are willing and available to help others.

> **Insider Tip:** If you are interested in learning from the experiences of others who have been on a search for biological family and want their help and advice, there are many places to connect with those who have been on a similar journey. This book offers some guidance but also includes additional information in the resources section to connect you to others.

One member of a private Facebook group posted these words of encouragement to those going through the search for their biological origins. "It's confusing and stressful," she wrote. "But there's also beauty in truth ... People do recover and become stronger because of it."

Chapter 8: How family tree building starts

This section describes traditional genealogy basics. Its relevance to your search for information will depend on how much you know about the family you are searching for. It may also be useful should you decide to pursue genealogy as a hobby even after you complete the family tree of your immediate family.

Experienced genealogists sometimes will be open to helping adoptees and others who need help tracing their roots. If you know someone who has conducted any family research, you might ask for advice with a simple question: "Where do I begin?" You can also use the information provided below to learn about the key components of genealogy research and apply it to your goals as you get started.

Family tree building

Before DNA testing became widely available, building a family tree relied solely on genealogical evidence. In traditional genealogy research, the genealogist starts by putting themselves at the base of the tree, and then builds the family tree upward. They document information about parents and grandparents using paper charts, genealogy software, or online family trees, and progress backward in time to great-grandparents, great-great-grandparents, and so on.

For adoptees, starting with themselves at the base of the tree and building it out by going backward in time is a difficult endeavor. You might not have names or other information about birth parents and do not know where to start looking.

Karen took up genealogy as a hobby and built the family tree of her adoptive family. She enjoyed learning about the history of her adoptive parents and grandparents and how everyone in her adoptive family had come to live where they did and marry their spouses. She considered their stories her own as well.

After she reunited with her birth family via access to adoption records, Karen also began genealogy research on the families of her birth parents. She built two sets of family trees—one of her adopted family's ancestors and one of the ancestors of her birth family—and she described both as feeling like her family tree.

Karen's interest in genealogy was strengthened once DNA testing came along, and she was able to extend her family tree research even further. DNA testing also confirmed that she had found the correct birth parents. Not only did they verify them as her closest DNA matches, but her close DNA relatives "fit" where they should.

As noted earlier, genealogists advise beginning a family tree with yourself at the base of the trunk. After that, you will need to start searching for official documentation about events that concerned the people above you in the tree (in other words, your parents and grandparents). Chapter 10 introduces another way of building your tree—one family upward and the other downward. This is one of many creative approaches adoptees have used to combine their adoptive and birth family trees.

Vital records

Vital records are a cornerstone of genealogical research. *Vital* has its roots in the Latin word for "life," and vital records refers to documents that serve as official proof of a life event such as a birth, marriage, or death. These documents provide information to help you record and verify the relationships between people on a family tree.

Not all vital records are created equal. Some will have more information than others, even if they are of the same type. Different jurisdictions have often used different requirements for the types of information included on a record. Some states in the U.S. gather quite a bit of information, whereas records from the U.K. or Canada seem sparse by comparison.

Vital records typically include these three pieces of information:

- The date(s) of the event

- The name of the person(s) for the event

- The place where the event occurred

Death certificate of Robert Denbo[1]

---

[1] Harrison Township, Harrison County, Indiana, death certificate no. 56 (1904), Robert Denbo; Indiana State Archives, Indianapolis, Indiana.

Birth certificate of Ralph Williams[2]

Some vital records contain additional information, such as parents' names or a mother's maiden name. This is important information to build out your family tree and help to determine family connections.

In the United States, vital records were not required in many states before the 20th century. Even if a city or town started to maintain vital records at an earlier date, the record-keeping may have been inconsistent. Also, many vital records have

---

[2] Liberty, Grant County, Indiana, birth certificate no. 633302 (1923), Ralph M. Williams; Marion Public Library Birth Index, USA http://www.marion.lib.in.us/request-genealogy-records-2/: accessed 2017.

been lost or destroyed over the years due to disasters and damage caused by fires, floods, and other events.

Overseas, the situation may be even worse. Even if vital records are available, access from outside the country may be difficult. There are also language barriers to contend with. If you must turn to vital records in another country, make a point of learning about the history of records and recordkeeping in that country.

One of the hardest vital records to locate is an adoptee's original birth certificate. While foreign birth certificates may be difficult to access for the reasons stated above, in the United States there is an additional consideration for adoptees, that of original birth certificates being changed so that the birth parents' names are removed.

> **Insider Tip:** In many U.S. states, once an adoption is completed, a new birth certificate may be issued. This amended birth certificate lists the adoptive parents as the parents of the child. The original birth certificate is typically enclosed in the adoption file which is then sealed unless opened by court order. Adoptee rights activists are advocating for change regarding this unjust way vital records are handled. Several states have, or are working on, legislation to change this policy making it easier for adopted individuals to receive their original birth certificates.

Non-vital records

In addition to vital records, non-vital records are important documents for researching family history. At times, they may be easier to find than vital records. Non-vital records include official records as well as religious records and other recorded information, such as:

- Census records

- Will/probate/estate records

- Church records

- Newspapers

No matter how good your research skills are, you eventually will reach the end of a line of vital and non-vital records. Figuring out the next generation back in time is not so easy any more once you reach that point. Genealogists refer to this end of documentation as a brick wall in your research.

Brick wall research

People who do not know their family history, such as adoptees, start out with what genealogists call a **brick wall**: a seemingly insurmountable obstacle you must learn to climb before you can learn about your past. You may run into several brick walls as you progress in your own search. Records might be hard to find, people may have changed names, or some other situation obscures the origins or history of yourself or a person you are trying to research.

Keep in mind that every researcher, no matter their experience level or family history, runs into at least one brick wall when building a family tree. Some may seem impossible to break through, which builds frustration and anxiety. It will take time and patience as you work on different approaches. This is especially true if you are an adoptee with your first brick wall being the identity of your birth parents.

Fixing common family tree mistakes

In the thrill of the hunt, mistakes in building a family tree are possible. It happens to all of us. Shannon traced the wrong Bennett family group for two years before finding a document that proved she had researched the wrong parents of an ancestor named George Bennett. How could this happen? It turned out that there were two babies born in the same town on the same day and given the same name, George Bennett, so the mistake is understandable.

Shannon's experience teaches a valuable lesson: Mistakes are okay as you are researching and tracking down people. What matters most is that if you realize you have gotten off course, stop where you are, then go back and try again.

Shannon was confident with her initial choice since the family stories and the records appeared to point her in one direction. However, after she studied George's siblings, and traced them forward in time, she discovered her error. This could easily happen to an adoptee, especially if you are researching a potential relative with a common name.

Below are some of the common mistakes made by adoptees who have done a search for biological family (and some tips for catching and correcting them).

1. Catching mistakes

Do not believe everything you read! Not everything in print is true, whether a book, a magazine article, or an online family tree. In genealogy research, new information is continually coming to light which may prove that someone else's hard work was wrong.

Before you solidify the people listed on your tree, consider creating a draft or a "working tree" which contains unconfirmed research. Create a paper or computer file where you gather information on the person(s) you are trying to prove for your family line and be wary of accepting others' research without double-checking their work yourself.

Always be skeptical of another person's research until you have completed the following steps:

- **Check the person's sources.** If that individual does not have any, treat the information as a potential clue, rather than a fact. A person with a family tree of many thousands of people large possibly did their work quickly.

- **Check the date.** Sometimes older information is better because it was still fresh when it was gathered. On the other hand, genealogists from earlier periods were often laxer when it came to documentation. Newer works that include footnotes tend to be the most trustworthy for current researchers.

- **Who was the publisher?** If the information came from a book published by a reputable source, such as the Mayflower Family books by the General Society of Mayflower Descendants, you can have more confidence the resource is trust-worthy and the data is accurate.

2. Fixing information that cannot be true

Be vigilant as you scour someone else's tree. If you discover a child in someone else's family tree listed as being born before his or her own mother, there is obviously a problem. If that tree is important for your search, it is up to you to figure out where the error is and fix it in your own draft of the tree. A basic best practice: If something looks unusual, make a note to follow up and be sure to follow through. If you have multiple possible dates for a single event, add them to your research notes. The problem could be a simple clerical error, or it could be the result of trying to fit someone into a tree where they do not fit. You might miss an important family member or clues about someone in the family that will be vital to solving your own mystery, so keep your eyes open for mistakes made by others.

3. Working with common last names

Say you come across the last name Smith. If that was a common name in the area where you were born and/or adopted, how do you know you have found the right family of Smiths when you start searching? If your potential family has a common name, you must take things slowly and methodically. Be extra cautious in matching important dates, locations, and connections to make sure you have the right family. It might take time, patience, and a whole lot of coffee. Go slowly and confirm connections with as many reliable sources as you can find.

4. Spellings that seem to change

When digging into old vital records and census forms, do not be surprised to run into multiple spellings of someone's first or given names (the name Arvin may be alternately recorded as Harvin, Harbin, or Harden, for example). Prior to the 20th century, the exact spelling of a person's name was not important.

In earlier eras, spelling was more fluid. Census workers sometimes guessed at a family name if they spoke broken English or they had to ask a neighbor for the information. There are instances where you can get a hint of a person's accent simply by looking at the way a clerk spelled his or her name on a document.

Chapter 9: Best practices for genealogy research

Some research into family history and genealogy can be done over the Internet. But not everything is posted online. Quite a bit of research will require making phone calls, sending letters, or even traveling to the location where the documents are stored.

If you are making a trip to look for documents or talk to people who may have more information, consider taking along a portable genealogy kit. It contains tools which help you to gather and organize your notes about what you discover:

- Smartphone for taking photos, recording interviews, and accessing genealogy apps. Get the apps and learn how to use them before you depart!

- Camera or portable scanner, if smartphones and cameras are not allowed

- Small paper notebook or electronic tablet

- Pencils and archive-safe pens

- Small ruler

- Sticky notes

- USB flash drive for backing up and transferring computer files

- ID/access/payment cards for libraries, copiers, etc.

When you are on a research trip, you will take notes—lots of notes! Keep your notebook or tablet nearby. You never know when you will get a research idea out of the blue. At other times, family may share a new piece of information. Often it is because the conversation turned in a certain way, and it triggered some memory. This is especially common when talking with older generations.

Genealogy researchers prefer to use pencils over pens because they are less damaging to paper records, photographs, and other items. Also, many archives, libraries, and other research facilities will not let visitors use pens in their research areas. If you do bring pens in your kit, we suggest you invest in a few different colors that use archival-quality ink. Unlike the acidic ink found in most regular pens, archival-quality pens will not bleed or damage paper.

It is important for you to think about how to keep your documents and other family items safe on the way home from your research adventure. Improperly storing your materials can lead to their demise. In the past few decades, a range of archival-safe products have come on the market, thanks in large part to the scrapbooking craze. Take advantage of them and ensure that you store your papers and photos in a way which will protect them for several more generations.

When you travel for research, also bring a sturdy plastic folder or accordion folder system with you. These are great ways to keep photocopies and other materials clean, safe, and organized until you return home where you can examine them more carefully. They will also not get creased or crumpled if you are flying.

Here are some general guidelines for storing and transporting papers, photos, and other materials:

- Invest in acid-free products (paper, document sleeves, boxes, etc.).

- Store large items in boxes in temperature-controlled locations (such as interior closets of your home, as opposed to attics and basements).

- Place documents in clear plastic sleeves inside of binders or folders.

- Always have multiple backups of paper and digital images.

Chapter 10:
Learning about genealogy and DNA

The goal for many adoptees who begin a search for biological family is to uncover their family of origin and the identities of each birth parent and grandparent. This requires **genealogy**, or the building of family trees based on available information.

Family searches that include DNA testing are conducted by people with specific skills. Most people can develop these skills given the time, interest, and dedication. Local genealogy societies, books, conferences, webinars, social media, and online courses can connect you with information that will help you learn how to search for unknown relatives the specific steps it takes to do it.

> **Insider Tip:** Making sense of DNA results and family trees takes both time and skill. You will need to learn how to navigate through an online DNA account, make sense of ethnicity maps and percentages, parse through the family trees built by other people, and learn to build family trees yourself. In many ways, learning to do a family search is similar to becoming a special detective where you must learn to piece together different types of information to figure out your mystery. If learning all of this seems overwhelming or impossible, you can work with an experienced search angel or genealogist. You might also consider asking a friend or family members to assist you or to do the bulk of the work for you.

Some adoptees have found creative ways to build a tree that includes their adoptive and birth families. You might consider making one family the branches of the tree and the other family its roots. Consider the way this family tree figure is structured as one example:

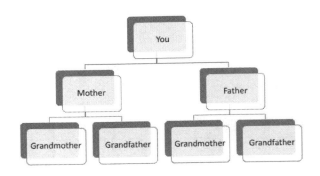

A basic family tree built downward rather than upward

The sections in this chapter will prepare you to think like a detective, get organized, and arm you with resources to develop your skills further.

Genealogical logic puzzles

Genealogists are like detectives. Working out puzzles and solving mysteries is their passion. Many genealogists joke about their addiction to family history research because it can consume a person's life. Late-night research sessions can leave you with a headache the next morning, or a few weeks later, when you come back to review what you discovered. This can be doubly frustrating if you did not take notes and have lost track of important information you came across along the way.

A paper notebook or a text document on your computer will work well to keep track of your discoveries. People who have experience using computer software often turn to spreadsheet programs like Excel or Google Sheets. Other people prefer spiral notebooks or binders. Whatever tool you use to keep track of your findings, it should be something that you are comfortable using and helps you stay organized.

When taking notes, try to include the following types of information:

- **Date(s)** research was performed
- **Books** or print publication consulted
- **Useful websites**. Bookmark websites you frequently visit, then create a resource list showing what they contain and why it is helpful for your research.
- **What you found**. Record what you did and did not find from each source, so you do not waste time returning to it again later.
- **DNA kit numbers and matches**. Learn and use screenshots in case information later disappears if someone deletes their account.
- **Surname list/location list**. Compile a list of potential family surnames and the locations associated with each one.
- **Correspondence log**. Record who you contacted, the information you sought, and what you obtained.
- **List of libraries, archives, courthouses, or other facilities** containing important records. Record the addresses, hours of operation, and other pertinent information.
- **Abbreviations and other terms**. Record government abbreviations, religious terms, and foreign words you come across during your research.

Insider Tip: When you are recording names, dates, events, or facts, it is helpful to take notes about the source of information. Was it from the family tree of a person you match by DNA? Was it from a family history website? Showing proof gives credibility to your work in tracing family. You may need to explain to others what steps you took to locate them, or you may wish to write about your experience some day. Taking good notes will make this possible.

Genealogy courses and conferences

If you choose to dive in and try your hand at genealogy and DNA studies, you might consider joining a local genealogical society if there is one in your area. These are groups of people who share a love and passion for all types of genealogy research.

It might seem odd to join a club of family history enthusiasts, but many members of these groups have decades of research experience under their belts. Some societies offer special interest groups (SIGs) that focus on DNA research. Joining a DNA SIG will put you in touch with real people who may be able to help you with your research.

Attending conferences and seminars is a great way to network with other people while learning about new techniques and research stories. A few of the larger national conferences are now live-streaming sessions for those who cannot travel to the physical events. Often there is a DNA track or classes offered on adoption research. A list of some of the regular conferences and educational seminars is provided below.

- **National Genealogical Society Conference:** Held in a different city every year, typically in May.

- **Federation of Genealogical Societies Conference**: Rotating cities, typically held in August.

- **RootsTech:** Every February in Salt Lake City, Utah and October in London, England.

- **Genealogical Research Institute of Pittsburgh:** Takes place over one week in June and one week in July. In addition, the institute often offers classes in other locations over the summer.

- **Southern California Genealogical Society:** Annual conference takes place in May in Burbank, California, and includes a DNA day.

- **Institute for Genetic Genealogy (I4GG):** A new annual conference dedicated completely to genetic genealogy, held in San Diego.

Webinars are a great form of distance learning and require no travel. While many organizations offer free online lectures to registered members, sites such as Legacy Family Tree Webinars offer online lectures for anyone to purchase or on occasion listen for free. Topics vary and cover everything from basic methodology to advanced topics.

Finally, there are many social media sites, websites, and online forums devoted to genealogy topics. Some have already been mentioned before and some are included in the resources.

Insider Tip: If you do not participate in social networks, you can still gain a lot of information online. Two websites worth checking out are DNAadoption.org (free) and DNA-Central.com (paid), both of which contain a wide variety of resources to help adoptees and others understand DNA testing and how to use the results to trace family lines.

Chapter 11:
DNA: the game-changer for adoption-related searches

DNA testing has been a game-changer for adoptees. When records regarding birth and adoption are sealed or falsified, DNA provides a powerful tool that can offer clues about family ties and ethnic origins. DNA testing has also provided some adoptees insights into medical conditions for which they or their children are at risk.

In recent years, adoptees have turned to DNA testing to get past brick walls. Other individuals can use DNA as well, including people conceived with donor eggs or sperm, people raised by a single parent or adopted by a step-parent, and individuals abandoned as infants or children (referred to as "foundlings").

DNA complements the search for biological relatives, but in many cases, it does not automatically reveal who a birth parent is. If your closest match is a cousin, for example, there are often many potential people in the tree who could be your biological father or mother. Because of this, many adoptees use DNA testing in tandem with traditional family trees and data collection to further their searches. These techniques will be described in more detail in later sections.

Each person's reasons for turning to DNA testing are unique. The timing may be unique, too. DNA may play a role at the start of the search, somewhere in the middle, or at the end. Some people use DNA as a means of tracking down biological relatives, while others use it to confirm a genetic relationship once a suspected family member is found.

Identifying your goals for DNA testing

DNA is a powerful tool. However, not everyone will feel the same way about testing. Neither should there be any pressure on a person to take a test for a reason that is not their own. No two people, adopted or not, are the same when it comes to weighing the pros and cons involved in DNA testing and making decisions about it.

> **Insider Tip:** DNA testing is not necessary in every case to identify biological family. Obtaining birth and adoption records, asking for information from adoptive family and family friends, signing up for mutual consent registries, and doing Internet searches for public information based on birth records or other documentation are all avenues to reconnect with biological relatives. If these approaches are sufficient, it may not be necessary to take a DNA test.

When incorporating DNA into a search for biological relatives, the chances of success depend on a lot of factors. At a basic level, people biologically related to you will have to take a DNA test, too, for your DNA test to be of any help.

These are common reasons people seek out a DNA test:

- **Ethnicity**: Where did my ancestors come from? Did my parents have the same ethnic background, or were they different?

- **Matching with DNA relatives**: Do I have biological family "out there"? Could I find them through DNA testing? Can I get confirmation of paternity for the man listed as the father on my birth certificate?

- **Health symptoms and medical risks**: Why do I have medical issues? Could it be genetic? Do I have a family history of a condition that puts myself or my children at risk?

- **Curiosity/self-identity**: What is it that makes me unique? What makes me like everyone else? What could a DNA test tell me that I do not know about myself yet?

- **Establishing truth**: "People lie, but DNA doesn't. Can this test tell me the truth, once and for all?"

Ethnicity

People's sense of belonging in society has an ethnic component. For some, ethnic identity is an aspect of personal identity and provides a feeling of rootedness in human history. It can create a sense of membership or belonging with others who share similar physical or social characteristics. **Ethnicity** can be of value to those who feel that they look different from family members or the communities in which they live.

There is also a feeling of mystery or "otherness" that some adoptees have described, tied to not having access to knowledge of basic information most people take for granted. Not knowing or being able to answer the question "What's your ethnic background?" is a concern expressed by many.

Ethnicity assignments based on DNA results is a controversial topic. Some argue that the process of assigning ethnicity labels based on DNA is not accurate since not all of our ancestors' DNA gets passed down to us. Additionally, the makeup of a person's ethnicity pie chart can change over time as DNA testing companies collect new data and update their models.

Some critics argue that testing creates artificial barriers between people and can entrench false beliefs about race. A related argument calls for the practice of DNA testing to stop, arguing that ethnicity should not matter. Even within the scientific community, there is debate over whether there is value to testing for and reporting ethnicity.

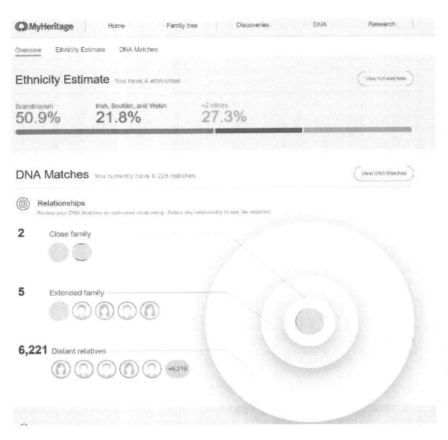

One example of a MyHeritage DNA ethnicity estimate

Ethnicity is a gray area and leads to spirited debate. Your perspective as an adoptee should be recognized and respected on this matter. Regardless of what anyone else might say, you might feel that information for ethnicity testing is personally significant, and DNA testing is a vital tool to understanding your history. Chapter 16 covers this topic more deeply.

Matching with DNA Relatives

Online DNA databases for genealogists have changed the way that adoptees and birth families search for one another. More adoptees are using DNA testing to look for biological family.

The process for getting started is easy:

1. Find a testing service that lets members compare their DNA results online.

2. Order a kit online or over the phone. Some services offer kits through Amazon and other online retailers.

3. Register your kit at the testing service's website.

4. Provide a sample using a cheek swab or by spitting into a small vial that comes with the kit.

5. Return the DNA sample to the testing service via postal mail.

6. Wait for an email notifying you that your DNA results are ready.

The testing services' websites have lots of features, but adoptees will be most interested in the DNA match list. This is a list of people who share at least some DNA because of a recent or more distant family connection.

Close relatives will share large chunks of DNA. A child gets roughly 50% of his or her DNA from each parent and will share between 7% and 13% of DNA with a first cousin. Distant relatives will have far less DNA in common. A fourth or fifth cousin will have only a fraction of one percent of shared DNA.

When your results are ready, you can opt-in to see a list of the people who are most closely related to you. Testing companies estimate how close you are related to each of the individuals on the list based on the total amount of shared DNA and size of shared DNA **segments** (chunks of DNA you and another person have in common).

Segments that are important are sizeable regions where DNA markers are identical between two people, most commonly because they have been inherited from the same parent, grandparent, or more distant ancestor.

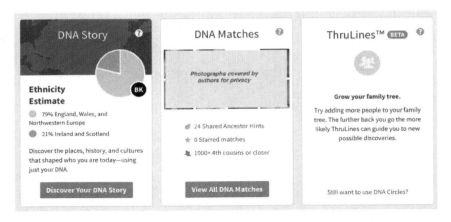

AncestryDNA report summary

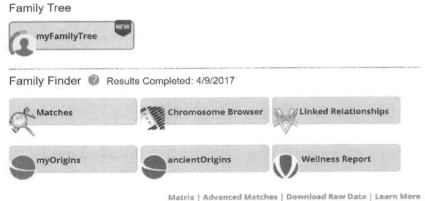

Family Tree DNA (FTDNA) report summary

Note: The appearance of the DNA results landing page changes over time as a company updates and changes its tools and reports.

The people on your match list may list their full names. Others may use initials (MLR) or screen names (JollyRancher66). Some matches may have put together family trees and posted them alongside their DNA results. Others will not provide any extra information about their extended families or reveal clues about their real-life identities.

> **Insider Tip:** The closer the DNA match (in other words, the more DNA you share with another person on the list), the easier it is to search through that person's family tree to figure out who your biological parent might be. The most helpful matches are usually second cousins or closer. Those with large and public family trees are the best matches to spend time reviewing because their family trees provide you instant information without having to take the next step of messaging or communicating.

The more distantly-related you and a match are, the more likely the common ancestor you share will be farther back in your respective family trees. For example, you and someone estimated to be your third or fourth cousin may share a great-great-grandparent or great-great-great-grandparent born in the 1800s. There may be hundreds of descendants to explore before you can narrow down the identity of a close relative.

The more distantly related a DNA match is, the more difficult and time-intensive it will be to use that match's DNA information and family tree to make progress in your search for biological family. You may have to investigate family trees with dozens or hundreds of people in it. Figuring out which person on a huge family tree might be your grandparent or a biological parent can be a daunting task. A way to overcome this is to continue testing at different companies until you have determined where your closest DNA matches reside. The catch with getting a match from one of these DNA matching databases is that someone related to you typically must have tested *at the same company*.

How quickly does matching happen?

Waiting on results after you submit a kit varies from one company to the next, but typically takes a few weeks to a month or two. Most of the work to match testers to one another gets figured out before you get notification of your results being ready. When you log in, you should have matches already there.

We have seen it take a few additional days after test results are available online before all the matches appear. This can cause panic if you do not match right away to someone you are expecting to, or if you have no close matches show up immediately.

Some people will find a close match right away, typically because the other person was already actively searching for them. Other people may wait for months or years for someone in their genetic family to appear as a match.

If after a few days of receiving your results, you find there are still no close or helpful matches, it may be that none of your biological relatives has decided to test yet. There is no way to predict ahead of sending in your DNA sample if you will get a helpful match, or how long it might take.

Why am I not getting any close matches?

You may open your DNA test results only to see your closest match is a third or fourth cousin. There are many explanations for having a match list without close relatives, and none of the reasons is your fault. Consider these possibilities:

- Your birth parents or close biological family members have died.

- Your birth family is relatively small.

- Your birth family lives in a different part of the world where the test you have taken is not available.

- You have tested at a different company than your biological relatives have.

- Your birth family relatives do not know about you, hence they do not know they should test.

Sometimes, giving it more time will result in a closer match popping up. Double-check that you have opted in to the relative matching feature at each place you test so that notifications are automatically sent to you if a new match appears. Continue to check in on your DNA accounts every few weeks or months.

What does it mean to "fish" in all the DNA ponds?

Genetic genealogists recommend an approach called "fishing in all the ponds" to have the highest chance of succeeding in your search for biological family. Put in another way, the more places your DNA is being matched to other people, the greater the chance you will find someone you are closely related to.

> **Insider Tip:** Ask around in online DNA search groups which testing company will be most helpful to those of your ethnic background or country of origin. For most adoptees, the best approach is starting with **AncestryDNA** (the largest database so far) and then "fishing" in the other company databases after that. Many people have found their most helpful match using companies with fewer testers, so do not discount any of the family matching databases until you have tried them all.

Here is one fictionalized example of extending the reach of DNA by "fishing" in multiple DNA testing ponds:

Jon decided to begin searching for his birth mother. Jon sent his DNA to 23andMe, but his birth mother Mary sent hers to AncestryDNA. Jon and Mary each learned about GEDmatch as another place they might send their DNA data. Mary transferred her DNA raw data (see end of chapter for definition) first. A few months later, Jon transferred his data, and soon after, Jon and Mary appeared in each other's list of matches at GEDmatch.

Fishing in all the ponds is an expensive proposition, so some people choose to test at one company at a time, or they make use of free or low-cost transfers to get the most out of the money they spend on one or a few DNA tests. In some cases, only one test is needed to get to an informative match. The section in Chapter 17 called "Getting the most out of your testing at the lowest cost" explores this topic further.

Insider Tip: The **DNA Detectives** have created a flowsheet which is available to members of their Facebook group. The flowsheet gives testers a strategy to get the most mileage out of their tests using the least costly approach. Check the resources section of this book for the link to join the group.

Can I use a DNA test for confirmation of a person I already suspect is related?

You may have already identified a person you believe is a biological relative, but you or they want confirmation of it by DNA. Genealogical DNA testing is a perfectly good option for doing this, but some people will want to confirm using a paternity or maternity test either because it is more private or they want it established legally.

If being pressured to not accept DNA as "true" results, understand that push-back and doubt are common responses especially when it reveals an unexpected family discovery. DNA testing for genealogical matching is reliable, especially for relationships showing close and immediate relatives. You may need to be patient and find different ways to explain this to those who are resistant. Part 3 will arm you with more details on making use of you DNA match list once your results are ready.

Health Conditions and Risks

Outside of its use for connecting biological relatives to one another, DNA testing can also provide health information. Because DNA is a molecule that impacts the way our body cells grow and function, DNA testing adds another possible layer of information for adoptees.

Every day, we learn more about genetic factors for medical conditions. Cardiologists are using DNA tests to identify the reason for heart attacks that run in the family, for example. Oncologists and others can use certain DNA tests to determine which type of chemotherapy or other medication is going to work the best for which patient.

People who are adopted wonder if they are predisposed to any medical conditions, and like everyone else, they are curious whether DNA testing could help them to learn more about their risks.

You may have children and grandchildren now or in the future and want to provide them with family medical history that they can take to their doctors. Which DNA test is the most relevant to you, and how do you get the right test for your situation? These are questions still being worked out in the medical genetics community, but the interest in testing for these purposes is driving the market of medical DNA tests ahead at full steam.

Karen, mentioned earlier in the book, was adopted as an infant. Although she had been able to gather partial medical history from adoption records, Karen did not connect with biological family to gather full history and had not considered doing DNA testing until after her third child was born with some health concerns. Doctors were unable to provide an explanation for her son's medical issues, which prompted Karen to seek out more family medical history.

After finding and connecting with both sides of her genetic family, Karen asked for and received updated health information. All of Karen's children and the future generations of her family now are able to give complete family health history at the doctor's office.

Many adoptees often have little or no family medical history, and some may not even have information about their own health from early on in life. The appeal of DNA testing to help fill in the gaps of knowledge is understandable.

Both DNA testing and family medical history are important for you. One does not replace the other. The last part of this book (Chapters 22-27) explores this topic in depth and covers both DNA test options and paths to family medical history for you to consider.

Curiosity/Self-identity

You may wonder what makes you different from or the same as those in the family you grew up with, your friends, or your community. Some tests promise to tell you something about how your DNA has made you unique. Curiosity is natural, as is the attraction to DNA testing that promises to give us insight into hidden aspects of ourselves.

A DNA test can satisfy curiosity about what makes us different from, and yet the same as, other people. Interest over our own unique DNA sequence often has nothing to do with other people or with health or medical concerns. Like one advertisement for the DNA testing company 23andMe says about its testing offering: "This is a story about why you became *who you are*."

Similar marketing for DNA testing by AncestryDNA has also aimed to pique curiosity. The success of these campaigns to reach people and encourage them to test has been dramatic, as this chart shows:

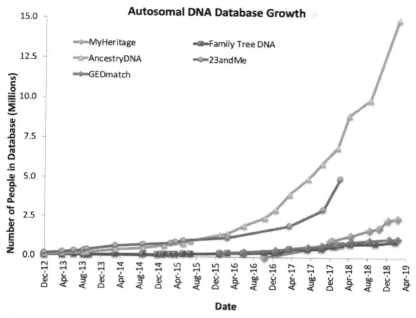

© 2019 by Leah Larkin, www.theDNAgeek.com/dna-tests

Autosomal DNA database growth[3]

Getting back results can be profound to an adoptee who may have had no biological tie to anyone they knew before testing. This can affect a sense of identity and connection with others.

Katrina compared being an adoptee to feeling like an alien. "You cannot imagine what it felt like to be adopted and then to do a DNA test and see pages and pages of people connected to you by DNA," she explained to Brianne. "I didn't feel like an alien who had been dropped out of the sky anymore."

---

[3] Permission for use of this graph was granted to authors by Leah Larkin, March 20, 2019.

Pieces of identity come together from how we view ourselves and our links to the people in our family, our community, and our world. DNA testing can add to and take away the bits of information we use to create a sense of self. Forming self-identity is complex, and results of DNA tests are now an additional factor for how this happens for people, including adoptees.

Establishing Truth and Preserving Information

DNA is no-nonsense. It allows you to bypass whichever people and systems are in control. As a result, you will hear "DNA doesn't lie" as a common refrain in genealogy circles.

For people who have had their biological origins erased by sealed records or stories that are subject to inaccuracies, a DNA test can be a path to reclaim a part of their history. In other words, DNA testing can be a way of peeling back the stories told by other people and getting to the truth.

Companies that offer to match you to DNA relatives typically require testers to opt in before they are matched to others in their system. After your results are complete, you must log in to your online account and actively choose to join the matching system to participate. Afterward, you are able to opt out at any point later, but you must take active steps to do so. Because of the opt-in/opt-out choice all testers are given, your ability to see who you are matching may change over time.

If one of your matches later decides to opt out of the matching database, or if they delete their DNA account permanently, that person will disappear from your list. To preserve the information once you have it, some people permanently record matches by saving to their computer what are called screenshots or screen captures.

Look up the steps to creating screenshots using the "help" section on your computer or tablet, if you have not done this before. Plan to store the screenshots in an organized system that will allow you to go back and find a person if they later delete their account. You might find that it works to organize the files by family name, DNA account user name, initials, date the screenshot was made, or another combination of information.

Raw data: what it is and why it matters to a search for family

We will talk about raw data at this point because this is a phrase you will come across often in the world of at-home DNA testing. **Raw data** is a computerized file of DNA information. There are different types of raw data files that can be produced by DNA analysis. For genealogical purposes, this typically refers to a VCF file, which stands for variant call format.

```
#AncestryDNA raw data download
#This file was generated by AncestryDNA at: 06/19/2016 20:18:45 MDT
#Data was collected using AncestryDNA array version: V1.0
#Data is formatted using AncestryDNA converter version: V1.0
#Below is a text version of your DNA file from Ancestry.com DNA, LLC.  THIS
#INFORMATION IS FOR YOUR PERSONAL USE AND IS INTENDED FOR GENEALOGICAL RESEARCH
#ONLY.  IT IS NOT INTENDED FOR MEDICAL OR HEALTH PURPOSES.  THE EXPORTED DATA IS
#SUBJECT TO THE AncestryDNA TERMS AND CONDITIONS, BUT PLEASE BE AWARE THAT THE
#DOWNLOADED DATA WILL NO LONGER BE PROTECTED BY OUR SECURITY MEASURES.
#WHEN YOU DOWNLOAD YOUR RAW DNA DATA, YOU ASSUME ALL RISK OF STORING,
#SECURING AND PROTECTING YOUR DATA.  FOR MORE INFORMATION, SEE ANCESTRYDNA FAQS.
#
#Genetic data is provided below as five TAB delimited columns.  Each line
#corresponds to a SNP.  Column one provides the SNP identifier (rsID where
#possible).  Columns two and three contain the chromosome and basepair position
#of the SNP using human reference build 37.1 coordinates.  Columns four and five
#contain the two alleles observed at this SNP (genotype).  The genotype is reported
#on the forward (+) strand with respect to the human reference.
rsid        chromosome      position        allele1 allele2
rs4477212     1         82154   T       T
rs3131972     1         752721  A       A
rs12562034    1         768448  G       G
rs11240777    1         798959  A       G
rs6681049     1         800007  C       C
rs4970383     1         838555  A       C
rs4475691     1         846808  T       C
rs7537756     1         854250  A       G
rs13302982    1         861808  G       G
rs1110052     1         873558  T       G
```

Appearance of a portion of an AncestryDNA raw data file

Raw data is important for genealogy purposes because it can extend the reach of your search for biological relatives. Like in the scenario with Jon and Mary earlier in the chapter, if you have tested at one company, you can use your raw data from that company to put your DNA in other databases as well, to extend the reach.

There are other sections of the book that describe "fishing in all the ponds" in more detail, but the main point to understand is that raw data makes this possible. Part 4 covers raw data in relation to medical/health and will help you understand the uses and limitations of raw data in that context.

Chapter 12:
Preparing for reactions and challenges

Common reactions

People react differently to an adoptee reaching out to connect with biological family. These following reactions have occurred in some families whether the adoptee reached out after DNA testing or a traditional search using non-DNA information:

- Some people have known about and actively searched for the adoptee and are excited and joyful to connect.

- Some people were not aware of the adoptee's existence and need some time to adjust to the shock, perhaps ceasing communications for a period.

- Some people develop feelings of embarrassment or shame at the implications of adoption for another relative (such as discovering their mother or grandmother had a child born out-of-wedlock).

- Some people delete their DNA accounts or reject all attempts at communication.

- Some people respond, but then try to create boundaries, for example, requesting the adoptee not reach out to a certain person or only contact them in a certain way.

A later chapter (Chapter 20) will go into more detail about what you might write in a message to someone who is a match through a DNA test. Communication between individuals and between family members is perhaps the most complicated part of what comes after the DNA test. Everyone seems to react in an individual and sometimes unpredictable way. Emotions can flare and lead to behaviors and comments that are not well-thought out. This can lead to both good and bad outcomes.

The reactions to an adoptee can vacillate widely, even when the news is accepted well. Here is one case in point. The gentleman in the following quote posted in a Facebook group that had recently found a daughter he never knew existed. She had been relinquished for adoption at birth more than three decades prior. He was happy to have discovered his daughter, but he struggled as well. He wrote,

> "Thirty-two years after the fact, I become a new father, father-in-law and a grandfather all in one day...What can I say? The emotions run from euphoria to dread."

The emotional experience before, during, and after a family search is different for one person to the next. The impact on each relationship between people in a family differs from one pair to the next. There are common experiences, but no singular one. Making predictions is nearly impossible.

Preparing for unexpected challenges

Every day, new success stories are shared through television commercials, online circles, published personal memoirs, and news articles. These describe family discoveries and sometimes in-person reunions made possible by DNA matching databases.

Although some stories highlight the difficulties and the emotional journey one or the other side goes through, ones coming from the DNA testing companies themselves tend to highlight only the happy parts.

Be aware going into the DNA testing journey that not every story ends happily, and it is normal if you or your biological family end up struggling. Not every family member adjusts to a new family member or new relationships forming in the family. Sometimes acceptance does come, but only months or years later.

Sometimes DNA testing leads to the uncovering of unexpected information, such as high levels of **ROH** found from DNA analysis. **High ROH** is a DNA pattern suggesting the parents of the adoptee were close relatives to each other. It is covered in chapter 21.

In-person reunions can lead to intense experiences and intense feelings. These are common and normal. Some people find themselves confused by an experience of genetic sexual attraction (GSA) which they may not have been aware of as a possibility or prepared for. This unexpected feeling of romantic attraction between biological relatives and sometimes occurs for family members who meet for the first time as adults.

These less-talked-about challenges require extra support, understanding, and help from someone who understands them. Online support groups formed for those who discover information after a DNA test that is upsetting or requires extra support and understanding to grapple with (see resources section).

Part 1 - Takeaway Points

- Options for progressing with an adoption-related search include: records research, mutual consent registries, confidential intermediaries, DNA testing with family matching, hiring a professional genealogist or experienced searcher, or finding a search angel, family, or friend willing to volunteer time to work with you.

- Identify your reasons for an adoption-related search and look for sources of support before, during, and after.

- Give thought to the emotions, the expectations, and the ethical concerns involved in a search and how you and others might react depending on the outcome.

- Gathering, organizing, and recording information helps build accurate family trees for your search.

- Genealogy can be a hobby you participate in whether you want to document your biological family, your adoptive family, or both.

- DNA testing is attractive to adoptees because it provides insights into information that is not available from other sources, ranging from ethnic group and family membership to health and medical information.

- Identifying what is most important to you can direct you towards the right DNA test(s).

- "DNA doesn't lie," and as a result, many adoptees find it helpful and vital to getting straight answers about their past.

- Some outcomes of DNA testing and post-adoption reunions are more difficult to understand and adjust to and have led to the creation of support groups.

Part 2: Bringing Science and Research Together through Genetic Genealogy

The first section of this book prepared you for the different places to look for information and how to find support to get started on your search for biological family. This section will focus on genealogical DNA testing, a key step in the search for many adoptees who have already tried other options in searching for biological family.

Try not to let the details about DNA testing overwhelm you. You will not understand everything in the first reading, especially if you are new to DNA or have not taken a test before. Keep this section marked as a reference and come back to it to read (and re-read) again later.

Chapter 13: Genetic genealogy and DNA basics

DNA testing has become hugely popular for people who have what is referred to as "unknown parentage" for one or both birth parents. Adoptees make up a large group of these individuals who turn to DNA testing to help uncover the identity of one or both birth parents.

Others in the group with unknown parentage include **foundlings** (individuals discovered abandoned as infants or young children), those raised by a single parent, those whose present biological parent will not reveal the identity of the other (most typically, the mother will not name the father), donor conceived persons, and **NPEs** (people who make a "not the parent expected" discovery). NPE is a term that evolved from its original term of non-paternal event and is also referred to as a misattributed parentage event.

Sometimes men and women affected by unknown parentage have some information about their potential parent(s), and some others know nothing at all about them. It all depends on their situation, access to documents, recounted stories from others, and previous work they have done to sift through available sources of information.

DNA testing can open wide the doors to these people's pasts. They may find matches to people quickly, or it might take months. Their challenge is to determine how they are related to DNA matches who may be close family or distant cousins. This section will help you understand how it is done.

Genetic genealogy is quickly becoming a reliable way for adoptees to identify and connect with biological family. The three tests useful for genetic genealogy purposes are **autosomal DNA** (which includes testing of the **X chromosome**), **Y chromosome** DNA, and **mitochondrial DNA**.

For most adoptees, autosomal DNA testing is the most important and helpful test of the three. Autosomal DNA (you may see this abbreviated in some places as atDNA) is the number one test on the market. This is the type of testing companies like 23andMe and AncestryDNA provide. With one DNA test, you can learn about your paternal and maternal families as well as your ethnic origins.

In this section, we are going to examine what autosomal DNA is, how it is passed down to you, and what a genealogical DNA test will tell you. You will discover that autosomal DNA is an excellent tool for unlocking your hidden past, especially when combined with traditional paper genealogy.

Genetic vs. genealogical trees

An important distinction to understand is that every person has two overlapping family trees for their biological families. Understanding the difference between them will help you interpret your DNA results correctly.

Your **genealogical tree** for your birth family is your family tree of birth relatives based on documentation (like paper records documenting births and marriages). The tree can be built on information gathered from records like official birth certificates and from oral family histories about family couples and their children and grandchildren. For adoptees, this information may be limited before you start the search for biological family.

The other family tree, your **genetic tree**, contains those who can be found to match your DNA. This tree is smaller in number than any paper tree you will create because few people test and because the detectable amount of DNA you inherit from great-grandparents dwindles with each generation as you look back in time.

Genealogical research into a family can help a genealogist or other researcher build a family tree back in time for a dozen generations or more, depending on what records are available to trace. Building a tree based on genetic testing (most commonly by using results of autosomal DNA testing) allows you to search only about 5-7 generations back on your DNA tree. Beyond these generations, the DNA segments you have inherited from grandparents and great-grandparents become too small to trace back to individually-identifiable ancestors.

There will be people in common on both a genealogical and genetic family tree. Thus, there are two types of cousins you can have based on these trees: genealogical cousins and genetic cousins.

Genealogical cousins share one or more common ancestors with you, but do not always share DNA with you. On the other hand, a **genetic cousin** shares DNA with you so that they appear on both trees. For most adoptees, you will discover genetic cousins first, through DNA testing. Those cousins may lead you to even more cousins who have not tested. Your genetic cousins may number in the single digits, but genealogical cousins could be in the dozens.

Some people are surprised to learn that even siblings can have different genetic family trees even though their genealogical family is the same. Take for example the following chromosome comparison:

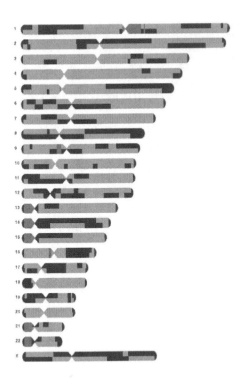

Family Tree DNA display of matching regions between siblings

This is a chart of Family Tree DNA's chromosome browser. Each oblong figure represents the chromosome pair for one individual. The differently-shaded segments display the regions of DNA he shares with a brother and a sister. The areas of shared DNA are regions of DNA inherited from their parents.

While these siblings share a lot of common DNA segments, you will also notice dark regions appear on the chromosomes. These are areas where the DNA the first sibling inherited from the parents differs from what the other siblings inherited.

It is entirely possible for a cousin to match one of the siblings but not all of them. This cousin might be a member of the genetic family tree for one sibling and only the genealogical family tree of the others.

Chapter 14:
What is autosomal DNA?

Many of you may remember learning about an Austrian monk and his pea plants in biology class. This monk, Gregor Mendel, is considered the father of modern genetics. Without him, and countless others who came later, we would not have made the leaps in science that occurred in the 20th century within this field. It was through scientific discoveries within the past century that we learned what genes were and how they were passed on.

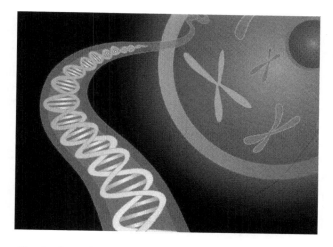

Illustration of chromosomes and DNA double helix.
Credit: National Institute of Mental Health, National Institutes of Health.[4]

Deoxyribonucleic Acid (DNA) is the basic building block of life and makes us who we are. Think of it as code a computer

---

reads to run a program. DNA is passed down from parent to child through chromosomes giving our bodies the instructions it needs for our height, eye color, hair color, and more.

DNA is a structure made up of sugars, phosphates, and bases which resembles a ladder when stretched out straight. Usually, DNA is curled into a tight little package within our cell's nucleus which we call a chromosome. The other type of DNA in humans is called mitochondrial DNA. This is found in our cell's **mitochondria** and has a circular, ring-like shape. Mitochondria and mitochondrial DNA are discussed in greater detail later.

Autosomal DNA is contained in the numbered (non-sex) chromosomes located in the nucleus of the cell The sex chromosomes (X and Y) are the 23rd pair of chromosomes and determine if you are a genetic male (XY) or female (XX). There are exceptions to the number of chromosomes a person will have, but most people have 23 pairs, or 46 total chromosomes.

Non-sex chromosomes, also known as autosomes, are numbered 1 – 22 and arranged by size. Chromosome 1 being the largest and 22 the smallest. The part of the DNA genealogy researchers are most interested in are the bases. There are four: Adenine (A), Cytosine (C), Thymine (T) and Guanine (G).

Bases pair up with each other, A partnering with T and C partnering with G, in what are known as base pairs. These pairs of A-T or C-G create the rungs of DNA ladder. Groups of thousands of bases connect to form genes which in turn influence who we are. It is these bases (the ladder rungs) that are analyzed by DNA tests.

Our DNA sequences came from our ancestors, sections of which we share with family members. By comparing our DNA to that of potential relatives, we can better determine our relationship to them.

Autosomal DNA testing is available to everyone, genetic males and females. At this point, it is the cheapest of the tests available for genetic genealogy. The average price for a test runs just under 100 USD compared to some tests that are 160 USD or more.

Companies Providing Genealogical DNA Testing

The companies currently offering the option to match you with other testers are*:

- 23andMe
- AncestryDNA (Ancestry.com's DNA test)
- Family Tree DNA (FTDNA)
- Living DNA
- MyHeritage

If you tested somewhere else, you could also transfer your autosomal DNA data to these places*:

- GEDmatch/GEDmatch Genesis
- MyHeritage
- FTDNA
- DNA.land

*These options can change, so at the time of publication, these were the available options.

The consumer DNA market is fast-growing, and the services and offerings will grow and change over time. You should check with online sources, such as the website of the **International Society for Genetic Genealogy** (isogg.org), for the most up-to-date information about your test options.

With all these options, you might wonder which test to choose. There are a few strategies you can consider as briefly introduced in Chapter 11. Here are a few more strategies to consider:

1. Test at AncestryDNA first, then fish in the other ponds if you have no close matches.

2. Test at AncestryDNA, 23andMe and Living DNA, then transfer a raw data file to GEDmatch, MyHeritage, and FTDNA in order to fish in all the ponds.

3. Contact a support group or organization for the country of your birth to find out testing company recommended for your geographical region/area of the world.

Privacy and at-home DNA testing

Some people have concerns about how their data is used by DNA testing companies and how it will be shared. You might want to consider some of these privacy measures and do more reading about assurances each company has set up regarding the security of your information.

- Set up a separate, new email account that you only use for DNA accounts.

- Order tests with a pre-paid credit card.

- Use initials or a user name rather than your actual first and last name when you set up your DNA account.

- Answer "no" to DNA storage and research participation if a company asks your preferences when you agree to testing (unless you know you are interested in these options).

- You may be forced to automatically opt in to certain features (like research participation) when you first agree to a company's terms of service; know you can later go back into your account settings and opt out of things initially required.

- Pay attention to DNA test company announcements about changes to DNA sharing policies and updates.

Understanding your autosomal DNA results

To use your DNA test results for tracking down biological family, you will be on the hunt for the closest DNA match or matches you can find. A **match** is someone who shares identifiable DNA segments with you because you have an ancestor or ancestors in common. The more DNA you share with a match, the more closely related you are to them.

The testing companies determine your matches based on the DNA you provide through your saliva sample. Each company has its own set of algorithms they use to cross-compare your DNA markers to other people who have already tested and are in their database.

These algorithms can determine how much DNA you share with someone. This is then turned into a list of other testers. The testing company also displays other information about your matches, such as whether they are genetically male or female and how much DNA you share with each one (often reported as a percentage or using a unit of measurement called a **centimorgan**, cM). A cM is a unit used solely in the measurement of DNA and is a relative distance along the length of a chromosome rather than an actual physical distance.

In addition to information about how much DNA you share, companies often provide a suggestion about how you and a match might be related. They might label a match as a close or immediate family (parent/child, for example). A match who has smaller amounts of shared DNA will be given a more distant relationship, like a first cousin, second cousin, or a range, like 3rd-5th cousins. The cousin range provided on your DNA match list can be vague, and it can be confusing to see and try to sort through when you first open your results.

During the weeks or months you wait for your results to come back, consider spending some time to get familiar with the appearance of the website of your testing company or companies. There are tutorials, YouTube videos, and blog posts you can locate with an Internet search that will demonstrate for you how DNA matching lists work and what they look like. Learn where the information about your DNA matches will be kept within your personal account page and how the information is displayed.

Once your results are back, you might see close matches or only have distant cousins. It varies from person to person and generally cannot be predicted ahead of time. A close match will make your search easier as you will not have as much work to do to figure out the identity of that person and how you are likely related. If your matches are all distant cousins, you may need to put more work into figuring out how you are related, and which matches will lead you to your birth family members.

A case example of family identification from DNA testing

The following fictional scenario is based on past situations and explains how information from a DNA match list can help in the identification of a birth parent.

Jack turned to DNA testing after finding out from his birth mother that he was conceived from a one-night stand. She did not know any details about his birth father except his approximate year of birth and the name of the university he attended. About a month after sending in his own sample to AncestryDNA and arranging a kit be sent to his birth mother, Jack received an email that the results were ready.

Following the instructions he read on a blog post, Jack logged in and navigated to the place on the home page of his personal account to click on DNA Matches. Up popped a colorful page with a lot of text. Jack searched around the page until he located the top of his match list. His birth mother was at the top, with a second match appearing right below her. This second match was listed under a box reading "Close Family" and showed a blue circle and a username. The words "possible range: close family-1st cousins" appeared under his username.

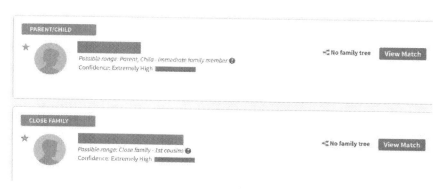

Display of a person's top matches at AncestryDNA to a female tester and a male tester. These matches turned out to be their birth mother and paternal half-brother. Note: The areas where a user name appears have been covered with dark gray boxes for privacy.

After checking on the amount of DNA they shared according to AncestryDNA's measurements, and messaging back and forth with the match, Jack concluded they were most likely half-brothers. Since Jack's birth mother had agreed to submit her DNA as well, and another tool called "Shared Matches" revealed she did not match the man who was a close family match, Jack was able to conclude this person was a match on his birth father's side of the family.

The age and geographical location of his match in Colorado seemed to fit with the story. Even though his birth father had not submitted a DNA sample for testing, Jack was able to figure out his identity by matching to someone else on that side of the family and gathering more information from AncestryDNA's tools and his match.

Not everyone receives a birth parent or close family match when they submit a DNA test. If you are one of those people, you will need to do more advanced detective work using more distant cousin matches. More advanced work involves studying the family trees of cousin matches to look for common last names, sleuthing for living descendants of possible grandparents using public information on sites like Facebook, Spokeo, and newspapers.com, and constructing drafts of potential family trees to try to fit possible ancestors and descendants together on one tree. These techniques are covered in more depth in Part 3.

Determining relatedness of a mystery person after autosomal DNA testing

Science is all about taking measurements and making conclusions with them. As mentioned earlier in the section "Understanding your autosomal DNA results," genetic genealogy relies on analyzing shared regions of DNA. Here, we dig into cMs a little deeper to help you be able to understand your DNA match results and use them more effectively.

Companies that report your DNA family matches measure significant pieces of shared DNA and add them together to tell you how much total DNA you share with a match, as a percentage or as a number of cMs. Some people like to work with percentages, and others find cM easier to use. It is a personal choice. If you prefer one over the other, you may have to do some research to learn how to convert one unit to the other because some companies only provide one.

Once you have information on how much DNA you share with another person, your detective work begins. There are charts of information that give the possible relationships between you and someone else, based on your shared DNA. The higher the percentage or cM value, the closer you are (and the easier it should be to determine how you are related).

Here are some examples of percentages vs. shared cMs for varying degrees of relatedness:

Percentage	Approximate cMs Shared	Possible Relationship
100%	6700	Self or identical twin
50%	3385	Mother or Father
50%	2640-3385	Full siblings
25%	1700	Grandparent, aunt, uncle, half-sibling,
		double first cousin
12.50%	850	Great-grandparent, first cousin, great uncle/aunt
3.13%	212	Second cousin
0.08%	53.13	Third cousin

Chart demonstrating approximate cM shared for given family relationships. Please note that this data came from the Shared cM Project created by Blaine Bettinger, and while the textbook percentages of shared DNA are fixed, the actual cMs shared vary for given relationships. The numbers listed in the middle column have been noted to change over time as the project collects more data.

The smaller the number of shared cMs, the further apart is the predicted relationship. There is ongoing debate about how small of a cM match you should consider accepting as a biological relative who matches you through a common ancestor in the past. Very small matches of DNA sometimes occur between people because of chance rather than a shared family connection.

As a rule of thumb, most genetic genealogists consider someone who matches and has a segment of at least 10 cM as a true match. Some will consider a 7 cM segment likely a real segment inherited from a common ancestor, especially if there is other evidence connecting you with them. Other evidence would be things such as paper documentation of how you are related, or multiple large segments of DNA that add up to be a significant amount.

Even though your DNA does not change, each company interprets your results a little bit differently. This means that if you and a genetic relative both test at two companies, there may be some slight differences in the shared DNA each company detects. Your total cMs shared with another person will be very similar from one company to the next, but they may not be identical.

Using a chromosome browser

You can also figure out your relatedness to a DNA match by doing an inspection of the graphical display of your chromosomes. There will be regions where you share visible segments with that person. Some companies provide a tool for you called a **chromosome browser** that makes it possible to see the location and size of these segments.

To understand how to use a chromosome browser to visualize shared regions of DNA, you should first learn the terms **Identical By Descent** (IBD) and **Identical By State** (IBS).

IBD means two or more people share an identical segment of DNA from a common ancestor and that segment of DNA has remained unchanged from parent to child. IBS, on the other hand, is when two people have matching segments, but the individuals DO NOT share a common ancestor. When this happens, it leads to many false positive results in databases when you are only looking at very small cM values.

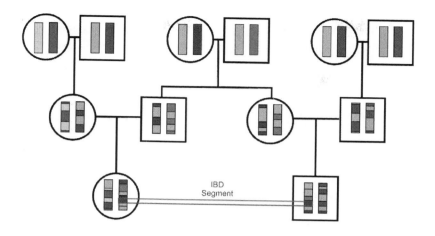

Graphical representation of an IBD (bottom level) to their grandparents. This DNA segment is identical because it was inherited from a shared common grandparent (top row, middle circle).

Fully Identical Regions (FIR) and **Half-Identical Regions** (HIR) are the last set of terms you will need to know when you are visually identifying segments. A FIR is a segment of DNA where you match on both the inherited maternal and paternal chromosomes. This is most common in identical twins, but full siblings can have FIRs because they have the same set of parents. On the other hand, an HIR is an area of the chromosome where one segment of DNA on either the maternal or paternal chromosome exactly matches another person.

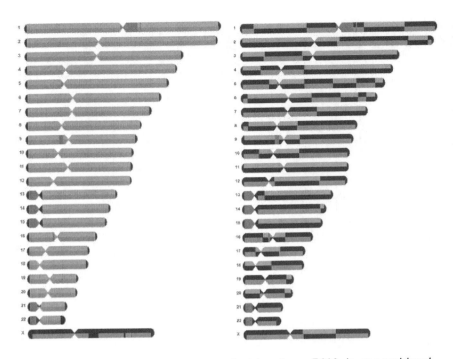

Chromosome browser images showing how DNA is recombined and passed from grandparents through a child to a grandchild. Image on left depicts a child compared to their parents, 50% from father (orange/upper half) 50% from mother (blue/lower half). You can see this child is male by the presence one X chromosome. When this child's DNA is compared to his maternal grandparents, the results on the right are seen. The divisions show how his mother's chromosomes are combinations of segments from the chromosome from her mother and the other copy of the chromosome from her father.

What is X chromosome testing?

Tucked into your autosomal DNA results is also the analysis of your X chromosome. Sometimes the X chromosome acts like a numbered chromosome. It matches up with the other sex chromosome, either X or Y. Two X chromosomes can share information, making them a window into some of the more hidden lines of your family ancestry. While the Y chromosome does pair with the X chromosome in cell division, it does not participate in crossing over to the extent the others do. Its most important role is to make sure that you have a complete and even division of genetic material in the cell.

The inheritance pattern of the X chromosome is unique, and it can provide a goldmine of information when you receive a genetic match on it. Due to the way it is inherited when two people match on the X chromosome and on other autosomal chromosomes you can drill down to a smaller list of potential candidates for shared ancestry.

Genetic males (usually XY) inherit their X chromosome from their mother. This X is a combination of the two X chromosomes she inherited, one from her father and one from her mother. Since a man only has one X, he passes it intact to his daughters.

Genetic females (usually XX) inherit one intact X from their father, passed through him from her paternal grandmother, and one X from her mother that is a mixture of X from her two parents. Females then pass on X chromosomes on to their children, both boys and girls. The percent of DNA you have in common from parent to child is shown here in the following chart:

Relationship	Approximate % X DNA in Common
Father and Daughter	100%
Father and Son	0%
Mother and Daughter	50%
Mother and Son	50%

Chart displaying the approximate percentage of X DNA shared between individuals in a particular parent/child relationship

Not all testing companies analyze the X chromosome DNA. There is hope that as the field of study grows, and as the users from these companies understanding of genetic genealogy continue to grow, more companies will offer these results. For now, the best company to test with for X chromosome DNA results is 23andMe. FTDNA provides visibility of X chromosome matching if certain criteria are met. Finally, GEDmatch provides an alternative location to look at X chromosome matching patterns between two people if a raw data file contains X chromosome markers.

How to look at the X chromosome and make sense of results is an advanced skill. You might search the ISOGG wiki and various blogs listed in the resources section for further instruction in making sense of X chromosome matching information.

Chapter 15:
Y and mitochondrial DNA

For family searches using DNA testing, autosomal DNA is the most helpful. It is helpful to all people, regardless of sex. Its reach extends through all branches of a family tree, both maternal and paternal sides. The X chromosome also adds additional information, as is described in the previous chapter.

Two other types of DNA, Y and mitochondrial, can offer some additional information in certain cases. Determining if you are descended from the same direct male ancestor as someone else you match is possible if you are a genetic male, for example, because of the Y chromosome. Determining whether you and a match both descend from a common maternal relative can be assisted by comparing mitochondrial DNA results.

Y DNA

The Y chromosome is the sex chromosome which is passed only from father to son. Unlike other chromosomes, the Y chromosome changes very little from one generation to the next. This makes it a reliable way for genealogists to trace a paternal line in a family tree.

The DNA of the Y chromosome can tell us on occasion which son from a common ancestor a male relative descends from. To be successful with using Y chromosome testing in the search for a biological father, you must pair the information from testing with paper genealogical research.

For genetic females, the search using Y chromosome testing is not possible, due to their lack of a Y chromosome to test. If you are a female and are in contact with a male relative on your paternal side (such as a paternal brother), you have the option of asking the male to test for you, to try to make use of Y chromosome testing.

There are some stories of success posted online in which males were able to accurately identify the last name of their biological father and his family; this requires having a special Y chromosome test available at FTDNA and learning about surname projects (see Chapter 19).

Using this type of genealogical DNA test may be a challenge if you are adopted and have only DNA information to rely on in your search for genetic family. To learn more about using Y chromosome testing to search for members of your paternal side family, we encourage you to join an online group or visit the ISOGG wiki (listed in the resources) to learn more about this type of testing.

> **Insider Tip:** Due to quality control issues, the raw data file of some people who are XX (typically female) sometimes include Y chromosome markers. This appears to be most common in AncestryDNA files from the version 2 (V2) test. There are extremely rare cases in which Y chromosome data in the file of a person who appears female might represent **microchimerism** (presence of body cells representing more than one DNA profile). Determining whether this has happened requires repeat testing with medical-grade testing, possibly requiring samples on different body tissues. Unless multiple, independent tests are revealing the exact same pattern, any Y markers in the file of a genetic female are likely a QC issue with the test itself and not microchimerism.

Mitochondrial DNA

Mitochondria are a part of every cell in the body and serve the purpose of generating energy for a cell to live. Mitochondria contain their own DNA, packaged into circular molecules. Cells contain dozens to hundreds of copies of mitochondria each with mitochondrial DNA. Women pass these on to biological children through the egg at conception; the sperm contain so few mitochondria that they end up essentially untraceable in their offspring.

Like testing of the Y chromosome, mitochondrial DNA testing has been available as a stand-alone test since early days of genetic testing for genealogy purposes. Most companies that perform autosomal DNA testing look at a portion of the mitochondrial DNA as part of that test. This allows companies to provide testers information about their mitochondrial **haplogroup**, a genetic population group of people who share a common ancestor on their direct maternal line. This can be powerful information if researching common maternal connections between close DNA matches.

The unique way mitochondria (and the DNA contained inside them) are transmitted through the egg at pregnancy conception makes it useful in tracing maternal lines in a family. If you opt for a mitochondrial test, learn more about some unique challenges involved with testing, such as heteroplasmy. **Heteroplasmy** is the term to describe when more than one type of mitochondrial DNA pattern is present in one person's cells, creating muddied results.

Like Y testing, mitochondrial DNA is helpful in some but not all cases of family searching. Visit the section of the ISOGG wiki dedicated to mitochondrial and Y DNA to learn more about how testing for these types of DNA may or may not be helpful in your own search.

Chapter 16:
Your ethnicity pie chart

We briefly introduced the topic of ethnicity in Chapter 11. Many people are familiar with commercials and television shows displaying people's ethnic backgrounds based on DNA using colorful maps of the world and a circular graph showing wedges of different ethnicities. This type of genetic ethnicity result is what many people go into DNA testing expecting.

Some people refer to this information as their ethnicity estimation or ethnicity pie chart. It takes on a few different names including ethnicity estimation, biogeographical ancestry, and admixture analysis; these are different ways of describing the same thing.

Estimation of ethnicity requires autosomal DNA testing. It may not provide any direct information about your birth family, but it can provide a deeper history of where the branches of your biological family are rooted in the far-distant past.

DNA ethnicity testing is important to many people in terms of a sense of identity and historical rootedness. An important point to remember is that these results are only estimates and they can change with time.

Reference populations

Your pie chart is created by comparing your DNA markers against those of current groups of people from around the world (called a **reference population**). The entire set of data from a group of people is called the reference data set and the people in it are referred to as the reference population.

DNA testing companies are continuously adding to the reference data. The reference population for Europeans is strongest in the U.S.-based companies at this time. Some companies have publicly stated they are working to improve ethnicity estimation for non-Europeans by seeking to expand their reference data.

Why ethnicity estimates change over time

As mentioned previously, ethnicity is merely an estimation. Because each company has its own reference data, your results may differ from one company to the next. You may also see your results change at the same company over time. This happens because each company compares your results against its own unique data set of markers from people around the world. They also change and update their analysis over time as new data comes in.

Here is an example of how one person's ethnicity results changed after an update to the analysis done by AncestryDNA.

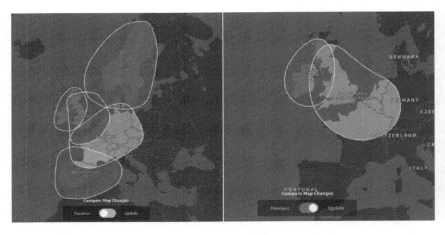

Screenshots of the same individual's ethnicity estimation using AncestryDNA's calculations before (left) and after (right) a 2018 update. Note that regions in southwestern Europe and Scandinavia appear to have disappeared after the update.

Some people have seen percentages of certain ethnicities go up and others go down. Small percentages (especially ones under 1%) have been the most likely to disappear from the results with updates over time. This is common and normal.

Some say to take the results of ethnicity with a grain of salt, but in some situations these findings have helped people look for clues and follow leads on their search for biological family. You may find it helpful to join an online group that focuses on understanding ethnicity results if you want to pursue this area further.

Chapter 17: Affording and ordering a DNA test

Once you have identified the type of DNA test you need, the next step is ordering a kit so you can provide the company with your DNA sample. For ancestry testing, testing is done on a sample you provide after ordering the kit online and having it shipped to your address.

The sample type requested will either be a saliva sample or a scraping of cells from the inner lining of your cheek. Testing on blood, hair follicles, and other body tissues are not available for DNA tests sold online at this time.

Detailed instructions for how to submit the DNA sample are included with the package that arrives in the mail. You can also locate videos online that will walk you through the process step by step. Before you ship back the DNA sample, make sure you register your kit by signing in to your online account with the testing company. Enter the unique code that came with the packaging. This will allow the company to track and link your DNA results to you. Make sure to confirm the email address you provide to the DNA testing company, so you receive the notice when results are ready.

Getting the most out of your testing at the lowest cost

The cost of DNA testing varies from one company to the next and from one type of test to the next. For most tests we have mentioned so far, the price can range from as low as 49 USD (during a sale) up to 200 USD or more. DNA testing can be a significant financial cost for some people, especially if more than one test is needed during the search for answers.

Some DNA testing companies will allow you to sign up and use their database of testers for free or at a relatively-low cost. Taking advantage of this cost-saving approach requires you to have a raw data file from another company that you can download from that company and then upload to another company's testing website. Review the section in Chapter 11 that addresses "fishing in all the DNA ponds" as a reminder of why it helps to have your DNA results in more than one place.

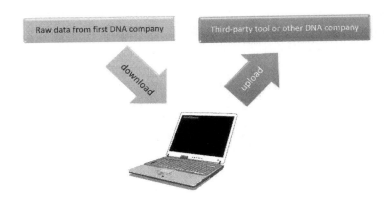

The options for using a raw data file to extend the reach in a search are expected to change over time. The ISOGG wiki and Facebook groups dedicated to DNA adoption searches can help you understand the process of transferring raw data files.

Kit donation programs

Some grants have been set up for adoptees to remove cost as a barrier to DNA testing. Some programs are specific to adoptees from a certain region of the world. One such program, called **325 Kamra**, enables Korean adoptees living outside the United States to receive free DNA testing. See www.325kamra.org/vetting for details.

The DNA Detectives accepts donations of DNA kits to make them available for free through their **Kits of Kindness** program. Other kit donation programs have existed for periods of time from private companies such as MyHeritage's **DNA Quest** program and a smaller program offered by the

Adoptee Rights Law Center, a legal firm that works to advance the rights of adoptees.

The ISOGG wiki has a page called "Free Testing" that is regularly updated. These free kits are specifically related to people wishing to participate in studies of the Y chromosome and specific last names, so they are generally restricted.

> **Insider Tip:** If cost of testing would otherwise stand in the way of you having a DNA test, you might try connecting with adoption-specific support and advocacy groups for information on kit donation programs. There are various types of programs giving away free DNA kits and these change over time as some programs exhaust their supply of free kits and other ones begin.

Part 2 - Takeaway Points

- You have a genetic family tree and genealogical family tree, and understanding the difference can help with a search for biological family.

- DNA testing for genealogical searching looks at the different types of DNA: autosomal, X chromosome, Y chromosome, and mitochondrial DNA.

- Autosomal DNA is the most helpful type of DNA to analyze for family search purposes, followed by the X chromosome.

- DNA companies outline how they might use and distribute your data in their Terms of Service and Privacy Policy documents.

- You can choose to opt in or opt out of certain extras like the matching databases, research projects, and long-term DNA sample storage.

- Understanding how each type of DNA gets passed from parent to child can help you learn how to narrow your search for biological family based on test results.

- Information about DNA matches can be displayed as centimorgans (cM) or percentages shared, or displayed on a colorful diagram called a chromosome browser.

- Ethnicity results from DNA testing can be interesting but will not reveal your biological relatives.

- The ethnicity pie chart can change over time as the companies update their reference data.

- DNA tests for purposes of learning ethnicity or matching with other people can be ordered online as mail-in saliva or cheek swab kits.

- There are ways to make testing affordable if it does not fit in your budget, such as applying for a free test from a kit donation program.

Part 3: What to Do After the Testing is Done

Previous sections have addressed preparing to search for biological family, gather information, and decide on which DNA test to order. These are important steps to help you gather information.

This next section prepares you to make sense of your DNA results when they come back. At first, this is often overwhelming and seems like a vast amount of confusing information. It was this way for us at the beginning!

It is normal to feel both excited and anxious while you wait for the results. Pause to collect your thoughts if you begin to feel overwhelmed, and start to get organized while you wait. By being proactive with learning and other prep work while you wait for your DNA test to process, you can hit the ground running as soon as you have your results.

Chapter 18:
Organize your DNA results

The most powerful part of DNA results for a person searching for family is the list of DNA matches. This is a list of people you share DNA with, the closest matches being at the top of your list and more distant family near the bottom.

If you do not get a close DNA match when you first test, you will need to start working with the DNA matches you have. There are different methods for searching through more distant matches, like cousins, to figure out how and where you might fit in their families.

Some of the tools to make sense of matches are company-specific, like shared matches and **automatic clustering**. Others tools are available at separate websites like GEDmatch, DNAGedcom, Genetic Affairs, and DNA Painter. Some techniques can be done using pen and paper or a spreadsheet document.

There are sure to be new techniques developed going forward, so check with DNA-specific adoption search groups for the latest tools at your disposal.

The DNA family member match list

No matter which testing company you pick, you will need to figure out where and how your list of DNA matches is displayed. When you log in to your online account, search for your match list under a tab across the top of your account homepage. It might be called "DNA Relatives," "Family Finder Matches," or something similar.

You can search the help section of the testing company's site, read articles or search for blog posts online, or find a video tutorial that explains it. Here is an example of the home page for DNA matching at 23andMe.

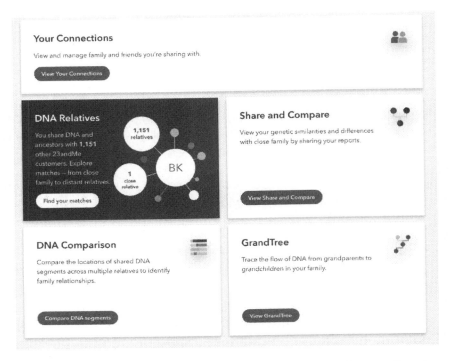

Display of the landing page of Family & Friends results at 23andMe. 23andMe occasionally updates and rearranges the information, so yours may not appear like this.

Once you familiarize yourself with the display, begin to focus on the matches at the top of your list. From the information available for your closest matches, you can begin to work on identifying and researching those people and their family trees.

You also can communicate with your matches to find out more about them, either through an internal messaging system at the testing company or via email if that information is provided. When a person responds to your message with information about their family, record that communication somewhere that is easy to go back and find later.

Once DNA information leads you to family trees, use the information on the trees to begin looking for clues about your biological family. You will eventually use the hints you gather to create a tentative family tree for yourself.

Creating and using a spreadsheet

Some people will organize the information they collect about DNA matches in a spreadsheet on their computer. The purpose of this spreadsheet is to organize information from your DNA matches to understand how they are biologically related to you or a member of your close biological family.

Examples of spreadsheet software are Microsoft Excel, Apple Numbers, and Google Sheets. If you have not created a spreadsheet before, you might search for some free online videos about how to use them. Most devices come with software already installed to create spreadsheets; if not, you can find free online options for creating spreadsheets.

Many people prefer a paper notebook or binder system for organization. If this type of organizational system works better for you, go for it. These are simply suggestions to help you get started. Feel free to use whatever system works for you.

Creating a Spreadsheet

In this section you will find an example of a spreadsheet created in Microsoft Excel to track DNA match information (names and details changed for privacy). This is only one of many different methods to track information, and you can use any system that you find works for you to track DNA matches, the amount of shared DNA, and other types of relevant information.

Username or real name	Shared cM amount	Possible relationship	Screenshot saved
M.S.	174	distant cousin	N
Dorothy Gattle	450	(half?) first cousin	Y
Robin Caruso	123	distant cousin	N
AncestorTrakr	1350	half sibling or niece?	Y
TJK1974	851	first cousin	Y

Example of a basic DNA match tracking spreadsheet used by authors. Columns include username or real name, shared cM amount, suspected relationship, and whether a screenshot of the match has been saved.

Some people create a separate document to track results from each testing company while others put the information all into one place. Either is okay. Keeping information separate grows more important if you have many DNA accounts to keep track of. You can always adjust your system of organization to make it fit your needs as you gain more experience.

Tracking your matches

Once your results come back you will have hundreds, if not thousands, of matches. Below are the columns that we have found work well for keeping track of the matches as we research them:

- Username for the match
- Match last name (if known)
- Match first name (if known)
- Email for match (if listed)
- Testing company where you match
- Shared DNA amount (percentage or cM)
- Maternal or paternal side match (if known)
- Date of first contact

- Match's suspected or confirmed relationship to you

- Most recent common ancestor (MRCA, defined later)

- Web address for their online family tree, if they have one

- Additional notes

Tracking DNA segments

Another piece of information you can track on your DNA matches is the segments of DNA you have in common. These are called shared segments and are described by their location on a chromosome. This is an advanced skill and typically used if easier methods of family searching do not give you all the information you need.

When you track a DNA segment in a spreadsheet, you typically will list the start and end points of a DNA segment. These numbers can be long (1 – 250,000,000) and many experienced users suggest that you round them to the millions. Segments are reported in units called Mbp, or megabase pairs. For example, 189, 234,110 could be abbreviated as 189.2 Mbp.

As you begin to study the details about the DNA you share with a person in your match list, you will want to add it to your spreadsheet or notebook. Below are the columns that you might add, to track segments:

- Chromosome where you have a matching segment(s)

- Start point of shared region

- End point of shared region

- cM for segment

- DNA letters contained in the segment

When you find regions where you and two other matches have segments in common, it can be a trail to lead you back in time to an ancestor you all have in common. The shared ancestor is referred to as your most recent common ancestor, shortened to **MRCA**. MRCA can refer to a single person (one grandparent) or a couple (grandparent set) that you and a person share. For example, 1st cousins share grandparents. Those grandparents are the cousins' MRCAs. Once you make a discovery of a MRCA, this can be added as a new piece of information in a new column as well.

Because AncestryDNA does not provide information on shared DNA segments between you and your matches, you will need to transfer your raw file to a different site, such as GEDmatch, to be able to use and track segment data.

If you have a close match or matches, you may not need to rely on this detailed type of investigative work to figure out your biological relatives. For many people, the family trees of their close matches and information about the close matches from their profiles or communication within messaging system will be enough.

Chapter 19: Tools and websites to help with your DNA analysis

Each DNA testing company provides its own set of tools you can use for making sense of your DNA matches, and these tools change over time. Some are extensive, some may seem overly simplistic, and some seem like they are the same from one company to the next but have small differences that can make a difference to a search.

It can be overwhelming to learn all these different approaches, but it can be done with patience and attention. There are numerous websites, Facebook groups, and blogs listed in the resources section at the end where you can go to learn more. Consider looking for extra support from others you meet in DNA search groups online, or from a family member or friend helping you with your search.

Here are a few examples of what you can use to make sense of your DNA results:

- A list of DNA matches in order of closest match to most distant (see chapter 18)

- A chromosome browser

- "In Common With" or "Shared Matches" features

- Automatic match clustering

These and other tools may change with time or go by different names, but they often have similar benefits to you, the searcher.

In addition to company-provided tools for analyzing DNA, there are more techniques and websites with online tools you can use. We review the clustering, phasing, triangulation, and surname studies next.

Clustering

The **Leeds Method** (see link in the resources section) is a way of color-coding your matches to look for patterns that help you solve the puzzle of how you are related to them. Some people find this colorful visual approach faster and easier than other methods as it creates smaller groupings. It allows you to look for patterns using color and to group DNA relatives into branches of your family tree.

User name	orange	green	blue	purple
Sar4519	tree			
Dan S.		▓		
Irina			▓	
ShaSha90		tree		
Jerod		▓		
LAgirl77			▓	
LeeJa			▓	
S.C.			tree	
HelenaFamTree		▓		
T.J.				tree
Zack K.			tree	tree
Gwen		tree		
DawnFTA			tree	
John J.				lg tree
Pat			tree	

Example of a Leeds method chart for a person's second cousin matches at AncestryDNA. Each color represents a grandparent or great-grandparent set that is shared for those within that group. User names were changed for privacy.

The creator of this method, Dana Leeds, has written about the approach in detail on her blog and website. There have been variations of color clustering developed, based on the original Leeds method.

Brianne's past two searches to find the birth parents of adoptees were successfully completed using only results from AncestryDNA and the Leeds method. Not every family search will turn out this way, but the development of techniques like the Leeds method and other tools that automatically cluster your DNA matches into family groups has greatly sped up the search for many people.

Other clustering approaches

A number of variations of clustering exist and like the Leeds method help to make searching through DNA match lists faster than ever before. You will see these approaches referred to as "autoclustering" or "automatic clustering" in some places.

The tools to do this work are available at a number of sites including Genetic Affairs, GEDmatch Genesis (Tier 1), DNA Painter, and DNAGedcom. Some of these sites are described in more detail later. Even the DNA testing company MyHeritage has made an autoclustering tool available to testers, and perhaps others will follow suit.

Blogs such as Kitty Cooper's (listed in the resources section) describe in detail the steps to use the tools on the sites mentioned above to automatically cluster your DNA matches into family groups. These tools will continue to change and improve with time.

Phasing

There are a few meanings of the word "phasing," but in general, it means determining from which parent, or ancestor, a specific DNA letter or region of your DNA came from. It might sound a bit intimidating at first, but with practice it becomes more natural and intuitive.

Phasing, most simply put, is the process of determining which parent (mother or father) contributed which DNA letter to their child at a specific location in the DNA. Phasing has limited use for most adoption cases since in many situations neither biological parent has yet tested. However, some success has been seen in using phasing, especially in situations in which one birth parent (typically the birth mother) has tested and can be compared against the adoptee. This can help in the search for a biological father.

Understanding how to phase your DNA results might lead to breakthroughs in your research if you have reached a dead end. With phasing, some people can often assign a DNA match to either their maternal or paternal side. Phasing also improves the certainty of conclusions you make about your results because un-phased DNA has a higher likelihood of representing or containing false positive results.

- The ISOGG wiki (see resources) lists some tools available for phasing DNA data. **The GEDmatch Phasing** tool is one place to do this work. You need to know the GEDmatch kit numbers for the parent and child (or other close family) who have tested. This requires a Tier 1 subscription in the Genesis version. (genesis.gedmatch.com)

Visual phasing is a specific type of phasing that focuses on the appearance of matching regions between DNA relatives, typically on a chromosome browser. It is defined by ISOGG as a "methodology for assigning segments to specific grandparents based on the crossover points of three siblings" and works when parents are not available for testing. This is an advanced technique, and there are other places to learn more about it. The Visual Phasing Working Group on Facebook is a group of people who share information about phasing relatives. (www.facebook.com/groups/visualphasing/)

Triangulation

Triangulation has a few meanings in the setting of DNA research. From the same root as the word triangle, triangulation of a common ancestor uses DNA segments. Using segment data from three or more people, you attempt to identify an ancestor of all three who likely passed down the shared DNA segment to all of them.

Similarly, triangulating a segment means you have found at least three individuals with that same DNA segment who have it because it was most likely passed down from a common ancestor in the recent past.

Successful triangulation requires the use of your paper genealogy research as well as DNA results so that the correct ancestor or segment is identified. As an adoptee, you may not have a family tree of biological relatives to start with. However, once you test you can use the matches on the DNA sites to triangulate segments. Essentially, you are looking for segments you and two other people inherited from a common ancestor.

> **Insider Tip:** Some of the testing companies we have discussed allow you to download your raw data as a .csv file. Where to find the file can change over time as companies update their websites and features. Do an Internet search for "how to download raw data" along with the testing company's name to find out the current way to find and download your data.

After you have your .csv file saved, you need to make the spreadsheet you are going to use for triangulation. It will ideally contain this type of information:

- The name of the person who tested
- Chromosome number

- Start and end locations

- Shared cM amount

- Relationship information

To weed out false positives and erroneous matches, you might next sort the spreadsheet by cM number and remove any matches below 7-10 cMs. This will give you more confidence in your matches and your final results.

After you sort your spreadsheet by cMs, run it through another level of sorting. Sort the spreadsheet by "chromosome" which will put all the Chromosome 1s together, then repeat for all the same start locations for the chromosome. The results will be an organized table with all of your matches grouped together by shared segments.

Now you are ready to start triangulation. Remember, the goal is to find groups of 3+ people who not only have similar DNA and ancestry but share a specific segment in common. If they do not share the segment of DNA you are looking at in common, they will not form a triangulation group.

Each of the testing sites you used to download your data also have resources to help you narrow down your possible groups for triangulation.

- **FTDNA**: Use the In Common With (ICW) tool on the "Matches" page to indicate people who share DNA with you and another match. This will not prove triangulation but will help you get started. The matrix tool is also great to help determine if potential triangulation groups fall on your maternal or paternal side.

- **23andMe**: Use the Family Inheritance: Advanced Tool to find matches that share common segments.

- **GEDmatch**: Use the one-to-one tool to determine if matches share the same segments.

- **MyHeritage**: Use triangulating tools and download a file of shared DNA segment data. You can mark your matches with an indicator icon if they have a DNA segment that can be triangulated with a third DNA match.

Surname studies

Surname (last name) studies are another way to attempt to understand your connection to your DNA matches and search through possible names of biological family.

Since last names are passed from a parent to a child (typically fathers to their children), genealogical studies of last names and DNA studies often overlap. The goal of surname studies is to show how all people with the same (or similar) last name are related.

If you come across a last name that keeps popping up in the family trees of your DNA matches, it might be a name you want to research a bit further. You are able to search for an existing surname study for many names. Some of these studies have results going back a decade or more. Joining an established study means that the connections you are looking for may already be there. Plus, you have access to administrators who can help you decipher your results as well as point you to the other participants who match you.

When searching for a surname study it is important to also take into account spelling variations. Just as you would look for spelling variations in records, DNA studies might also be set up under a name variation. Sometimes they list all known name variations in their title, which makes it easier for you to locate, but not always.

FTDNA has the most surname studies to date. Luckily you do not have to be a member of FTDNA to search their list of study names. Simply go to their home page and click their "projects" tab. This will take you to the page of current surname studies at FTDNA. You will learn about the project, who is accepted into it, what tests they require, plus any other information the project thinks you should know.

Cyndi's List (cyndislist.com) is a free website consisting of thousands of useful genealogical website links, including links to surname studies. The main page is broken down by alphabetical listings of surnames and resources. Simply click on the letter for the surname you are interested in and it will take you to the list of links. Beyond using a search engine to find a surname study, this should be one of the first places you should look.

For adoptees, surname studies are not the most helpful. But they might aid in a search if possible surnames of your birth father have been identified but you have not yet figured out the individual himself.

Third-party sites

Third-party sites are operated separately from the testing companies. To use these sites, you must transfer a raw data file there. Most are free, but a few operate by donation or for a small subscription fee.

If you find yourself needing to search beyond your matches at your testing company or to use tools the company does not provide, look into third-party sites. Note that once you transfer your raw data file out of a company's database, the security of your data is no longer guaranteed by the testing company.

Insider Tip: Regarding privacy, many testers create screen names or use initials when setting up their accounts. If you are concerned about privacy you might want to consider these options. Pseudonyms are not ideal as they can confuse and lead other family tree researchers astray. To further increase your privacy, you might wish to create an email address that you only use for testing sites, not for general emailing purposes.

DNAGedcom

The website DNAGedcom (dnagedcom.com) also has a few great tools to get you started. This website was first created by genetic genealogists who were helping adoptees searching for birth parents. This site allows users who have tested at multiple companies to upload their data into one place and begin further analysis using tools on the site. If you have already joined and use GEDmatch, you can also upload files from there to DNAGedcom.

The tools available to you at DNAGedcom are more advanced than standard ones provided by DNA testing companies. A few we have found useful include:

- **JWorks**: an Excel-based tool that combines the results from the major testing companies for streamlined analysis.

- **KWorks**: a tool that runs on your browser and will sort and group results from chromosome browsers.

- The **Autosomal DNA Segment Analyzer** (ADSA): a tool that creates a table for each chromosome with information on each segment though color-coded graphics.

GEDmatch Genesis

In the fast-paced world of genetic genealogy, you will hear a lot of discussion about GEDmatch. GEDmatch is like a matchmaking service for all your possible cousin connections, no matter which DNA testing company they used. It helps by extending your access to additional matches you might not otherwise have seen if you only look at matches provided by your DNA test company.

You will come across references to both GEDmatch and Genesis when reading about raw data file transfers. These refer to the same thing. The classic GEDmatch was the original site. GEDmatch Genesis was launched in the fall of 2018 and became the default site in February 2019.

To use GEDmatch, you must download a raw data file from a company where you have already tested. There are detailed instructions you can find online that walk you through the process of downloading your file and uploading it to GEDmatch. There is no cost to use GEDmatch, unless you want to pay for some extra tools.

Registering to use the site is straight forward. If you are concerned about privacy you have the option to also enter an alias that will be used instead of your name or to set your kit as "research," making it invisible to others. Note that you must enter your complete name for verification purposes by the administrators of the website. If you choose to use an alias, your name will not be seen.

Insider Tip: You may have heard of GEDmatch, as it is the genetic genealogy website that has led to the arrests of suspects in criminal investigations, such as the Golden State Killer case. Authorities are now also using the database at FTDNA to aid in identification of criminal suspects and crime victims. Some people feel comfortable knowing their DNA match data may be used by law enforcement to assist in these searches. Others do not want their data used for these purposes. There are ways to keep your DNA in these databases but exclude them from user searches by changing the opt-in settings or listing the DNA kit as research-only. No matter which group you fall into, know that your decision to participate or not participate is okay. GEDmatch and FTDNA are two ways to search for matches and biological family, but they are not the only way.

New GEDmatch users will want to check out the "Learn More" section on the main page. Here you will have access to discussion forums and learning sites. The forums are a great way to get answers to your questions. Adoptee-specific forums bring users into contact with others who have similar goals and needs.

After uploading a raw data file to your GEDmatch account, it may take several days for your data to finish processing. If you use the platform during peak hours, there may be a longer wait for analysis than if you use it during off hours. While there is no fee to use the site, donations are accepted which help with site maintenance and storage. This site can be used freely but a suggested donation of around 10 USD a month allows you access to extra features.

Finding success with advanced tools

In this chapter, we covered some of the websites, tools, and techniques that help with a DNA search for biological family. You might read about additional techniques not covered here, such as lucid charts, "quick and dirty" trees, and mirror trees. More helpful tools include the DNA Painter website which contains, among other things, the Shared Centimorgan Project relationship prediction tools (see resources section for link).

It is not possible to go into all of the details of each tool. Genetic genealogy groups and sites listed in the resources section are full of additional information. These places can lead you to the most up-to-date information.

It takes time and practice to learn how DNA works, and each search requires its own approach. Work with others who have experience with successful family searches to help yours go more smoothly and help you stick to it if you become overwhelmed or frustrated.

Chapter 20: Reaching out to your DNA matches

Making use of DNA match results relies on family trees your matches have built. Not everyone has built a family tree or posts their family tree publicly. This means you will need to reach out and try to communicate with some of your DNA matches to figure out how you might fit into their family tree.

You might be unsure what to say to encourage a match to respond to your message. In fact, it might be a terrifying thought, reaching out to a stranger and not knowing what to write and whether they will respond or ignore you. You might worry that what you say will make or break your chances at getting any helpful information. This chapter will arm you with ideas and advice so you can feel confident that you have given yourself the best chance.

> **Insider Tip:** Before reaching out to a DNA match, save all of the information you have about them. Either take a screenshot or write down the information, then reach out. Some people panic and take down their profile or delete their account when they realize they may have uncovered a family secret or happened into the middle of a situation involving others in the family.

Good news is that it is possible to open up the lines for communication and create trust from the first message. It does not take much, perhaps just a few sentences. You might be more likely to get a response if you are succinct and focus on being clear with your questions. An adoptee Lynne advised, "Approach your DNA matches politely and don't expect them to respond promptly if at all. Be nice and don't be demanding!"

Giving the other person something specific to answer is often the best way to open the door to further communication down the line. Your message when you first reach out should include:

- **Who** you are
- **What** you are seeking
- **How** to contact you (email, phone, through internal messaging system, etc.)

Here are some other considerations to keep in mind as you draft a message:

- Be **concise.** You can always follow up with more details later.
- Share briefly what you **already know** and what you do not.
- Be **warm** in your communications but also **authentic**.
- Acknowledge the other person's **potential emotional reaction**. Create a sense of safety and space/time for them to have that reaction.
- Communicate a balance of **urgency and patience** that fits your situation. If you need family medical history immediately, it is okay to say so.
- Consider explaining what you are **not seeking**. If you need only information and are not expecting further communications after that, feel free to include this.
- Leave **multiple ways** for them to reach back out to you, such as email, postal mail, phone and text.

You may need to send a few messages or wait for a match to finally decide to check their messages. Some people go weeks, months, or years between account logins. If you must send multiple messages to get a response, try to be reassuring about your intentions.

Some people who receive messages from a person they do not know believe it is a scam. These situations can be tricky to overcome. Be willing to give the other party more time, but rather than waiting on one person, consider moving on to the next closest match. You may wish to copy and paste the same message to multiple people at the same time to make good use of your time and increase the odds at least one of them writes back.

Here are some sample messages you might send to a DNA match:

> *Example 1: Hello, I see your DNA account (include user name) matches mine. Would you be willing to share your tree? I am researching how I may connect to my DNA matches and would be glad to tell you more if you're interested.*

> *Example 2: Hello, I see your DNA account [include user name] is listed as close DNA family. I think I have an idea for how we might be related, and it might be a sensitive topic for family. Would you be open to communicating with me about how we are related?*

> *Example 3: Hello, I am searching for information related to my biological family and I think you might be able to help. Would you consider helping me in my search? I'm primarily seeking family medical history and do not have any desire to disrupt a family or relationships. I'm willing to be discreet and hope you will be willing to help me.*

> *Example 4: We are a DNA match and from what I know so far, I think I may be related to [include user name] through my paternal side. I am adopted and trying to figure out and clarify who I am related to. Do you have any information or a family tree you would be willing to share with me to help me in my search?*

> **Insider Tip:** In your first message to someone, make sure to include the username, initials, or name of the specific DNA tester you are matching. Some people manage the tests for multiple family members, and they may not know which one you are matching.

You might want to have a trusted family member or friend review what you have written before you send it. They may have thoughts on wording and can be an extra set of eyes to check for grammar and spelling before you hit send. A first impression can be an important one to make when trying to encourage a DNA match to write back.

There are additional templates you can find from search angels and adoption search groups, if you need more ideas or want an outline for a longer letter or message. The Facebook groups listed in other parts of the book and resources would be a good place to start.

Try to put yourself in the shoes of the person you are messaging and think about what would encourage you to respond. Make it as easy and comfortable for them as possible by offering to use the messaging system, phone, email, text, or postal mail.

Sending a follow-up message

How long should you wait between messages? Every situation is different. When you email or send a message through a DNA company's messaging system, you have no way of knowing whether or how soon it will be seen by the recipient. You also have no way of knowing whether they will respond right away, take time to process it, or delete it without a second thought. All of these situations are known to have happened.

Two weeks seems like a reasonable length of time to wait between a first message and a second. If the first message was simply overlooked, this creates a backup opportunity for it to be seen again. Two weeks is also a common time frame for initial shock to wear off, meaning your second message might be received better. Know that this is a highly individual matter, and it is impossible to predict reactions of a person who is a stranger to you and may or may not be aware of your existence.

Some search angels avoid making contact and recommend testers avoid contact around the major holidays. These can be stressful times for some families, and some people have vacations or travel planned. This is not a hard and fast rule, though.

Anticipating varied reactions

Brianne and Shannon have worked with friends, family, clients, and DNA matches who were adopted and wanting to communicate with DNA relatives. While some messages have been returned, others have been ignored or not seen. For the most part, the responses from DNA relatives could be described as helpful and positive. Not every situation will turn out this way, but as more people grow familiar with DNA testing from media coverage, there seems to be less skepticism and negativity.

A friend from Brianne's community named June (whose story was introduced in chapter 7) decided to use DNA testing to search for biological family. June was 87 years old when she sent in her first DNA test. Using shared matches and family trees at AncestryDNA, Brianne identified both birth parents for June on the same day. This all happened shortly before Christmas in 2018. June and Brianne agreed to reach out to relatives on both sides of the family at the same time, using the AncestryDNA messaging system and email.

The reactions were different for the different relatives contacted, but the response was overwhelmingly positive. Neither side had any family members who were aware of June's existence, but most reacted positively to the news. One

DNA match quickly deleted their account without communicating, but all other relatives on that side of the family responded. The first response came back within 24 hours.

Communication has continued since then, and emails and letters quickly turned into phone calls and Skype sessions. One elder family member who is from June's generation has declined contact with the rest of the family for many years, and the appearance of June has not changed this to this point.

Within months of connecting with her biological relatives, June was invited to a summer family reunion. She will be meeting biological relatives for the first time in her life, six months after first discovering the identity of her birth parents.

It was a risk to reach out, especially shortly before a major holiday, and not every story will turn out as June's did. But it is common that adoptees will encounter different reactions from biological family. Some will choose to respond and will open the door to communications. Others do not extend such a warm welcome.

Preparing for the full spectrum of possible reactions

We covered briefly in Chapter 1 the topic of preparing for reactions from those you reach out to. The spectrum ranges from positive response to apathy to negative response. Try to consider the best outcome you could imagine and also the worst one; working with an adoption-competent counselor might be worthwhile for you leading up to the decision to make contact. If you are not prepared for the full spectrum of possible reactions, it might be best to wait for a future time to make contact, when you feel that you are.

Reaching out to DNA matches takes a lot of courage. It is risky to place yourself in a vulnerable position and not know whether you might be welcomed, ignored, or attacked. If you choose to reach out, be open to what comes next and know there are other people who have been in your shoes who can support you afterward, no matter the outcome.

Family dynamics are tricky, and some people you reach out to might need some extra time or need an opportunity to build trust to be comfortable communicating with you. Try not to read into the passage of days, weeks, or months as a sign the other person will never respond. The delay between messages might be explained by them trying to find a time to speak with other family members first, to figure out the circumstances and family involved in your adoption. They might even be going through a rough patch in their own life that has nothing at all to do with you.

Chapter 21: "Are your parents related?" and ROH

On the GEDmatch website is a tool called "Are your parents related?" (AYPR).

This tool was developed to look for signs of a specific pattern in the DNA called runs of homozygosity (ROH). ROH is a stretch of DNA markers that are identical for that region inherited from the mother and also from the father.

Looking for ROH in the DNA file of a person is helpful for genealogy purposes because it can show that ancestors belonged to a group that was endogamous (marrying and having children within members of a small and often isolated group). Examples include the Amish, Hutterite, Ashkenazi Jews, Acadians, and Polynesians.

DNA Applications:

- One-To-Many Beta - give it a try
- One-To-Many DNA Comparison Result
- One-to-One Autosomal DNA Comparison
- One-to-One X-DNA Comparison NEW
- Admixture (heritage)
- Admixture / Oracle with
  Population Search NEW
- People who match both,
  or 1 of 2 kits NEW
- DNA File Diagnostic Utility
- Are your parents related? Beta
- 3-D Chromosome Browser Beta

This screenshot shows how GEDmatch Genesis tools are listed. The ROH analysis tool called Are your parents related? (AYPR) is listed near the bottom.

High ROH: a special concern for some adoptees

An unintended consequence of looking for ROH means some people are now making surprise discoveries about their own conception. AYPR is able to detect if a person has been conceived from a mother and father who are close relatives to one another. This might be a situation in which the father and mother were brother/sister, father/daughter, mother/son, or another close relationship.

AYPR compares the similarity of DNA inherited from a person's biological father and biological mother. The areas of similarity and difference are displayed in bright colors on a chart of all of the chromosomes. At the bottom of the chromosome chart is information about shared amounts of DNA between the two chromosomes. It also states whether the tool found evidence (or no evidence) of relatedness between the parents of the person whose DNA test was analyzed.

When the DNA similarity continues over long stretches over many chromosomes, this discovery is referred to as high ROH. The numbers themselves cannot reveal the exact relationship between a person's parents, but with more data being collected, we are getting a general sense of the more likely relationships. ROH is highest for a child born to a parent/child couple, followed by a brother/sister pair, followed by other family relationships (uncle/niece, for example).

There is overlap seen between the various mother/father relationships that lead to high ROH in their child, so more evidence is often needed to determine how the parents were related. In some situations, a mother has revealed that there were sexual relations between herself and a particular male relative (brother, father, grandfather, uncle, or cousin) when told about the discovery.

If the mother is not available or is unwilling to discuss it, another way to find out is by testing the DNA of other family members (such as first cousins or siblings). You can compare these other family members' results to the person with high ROH using other DNA analysis tools, to rule in and rule out possible fathers.

GEDmatch provides contact information at the bottom of the AYPR results for CeCe Moore if you have questions about your ROH results.

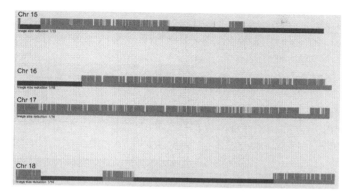

The dark bars (which appear blue on a screen/device) represent long segments of ROH across multiple chromosomes for a person whose father and mother were siblings (a brother and sister). Because of the amount of ROH present, it is considered a high ROH finding.

David Pike's ROH tool

Another free set of tools (developed by David Pike) includes an ROH analyzer. The AYPR results page links directly to this site. You are able to upload the raw data file you have put into GEDmatch and run through David Pike's utility without much additional work. The results of this tool are not as intuitive as AYPR.

If you wish you can use it as a second analysis. You may want to seek out someone who can interpret the results for you, or you can attempt to decode it yourself. There are no instructions available on the site at this time to help you understand how the ROH information is displayed.

Adjusting to the high ROH discovery

The discovery of high ROH is happening for individuals of all ages. At-home DNA tests are revealing this, and so are tests ordered in medical genetics clinics. If it happens to you, the discovery can come as quite a shock.

It is not discussed often or openly, but hundreds and possibly thousands of people each year learn that they have high ROH. The exact numbers are not known. Since this discovery is often made incidentally, there are likely many people who have high ROH and are entirely unaware at this point.

If you are doubtful of the results, DNA testing in a medical genetics clinic can evaluate and assess whether (and how much) ROH is present. A second independent at-home DNA test also could provide you a second opinion.

There are resources and a support group that have come together for those with high ROH. Search the website WatershedDNA.com using the term High ROH to find a brochure and blog posts on the topic.

If you discover high levels of ROH in your DNA using the AYPR tool, you might wish to change the settings on your kit at GEDmatch to "research." This will keep your kit number and analysis protected from the view of others.

Unexpected information can be hard to accept, especially if involves deep stigma or a taboo like sex between family members. Even though no one is at fault and none of us has a say in the circumstances of our own conception, it can be difficult to learn your parents were related to one another. Seek out support if you are struggling with your ROH discovery. Know there is a tight-knit community that understands what you are going through right now.

Part 3 - Takeaway Points

- Spreadsheets and other organization systems you create will help you keep track of information on your DNA test(s) and DNA matches.

- Tools to analyze DNA results include those provided by the testing companies and those created by independent third parties.

- GEDmatch is the most common third-party site for genealogical DNA analysis out there, but always be on the lookout for new ones.

- You can find a lot of support and information online if you run into issues or are confused by the analysis tools provided by companies and third parties.

- You can learn how to use these tools and techniques from free online groups and paid memberships to DNA learning groups.

- If you have identified potential lines of your biological father, participating in surname projects could help.

- There are templates available for what to include in a message to a DNA match, if you need help figuring out what to say.

- Anticipating the reaction of people you reach out to can be near impossible, but there are things you can do to increase your chances of being well-received.

- High ROH is an unexpected discovery some adoptees make when they use the "Are your parents related?" tool at GEDmatch; resources and support are available.

Part 4: DNA Tests and the Search for Health Information

Family history is more than the story of ancestors. Family history also includes medical information and details about family member causes of death.

People who are raised by genetic relatives often take their family health history for granted. Many adoptees are at a disadvantage from not having ongoing contact or even basic access to information about their biological family.

Tests designed for genealogical searching—the ones that the earlier sections of the book have addressed—were not created to be medical tests. Medical-grade DNA tests have more thorough coverage across stretches of DNA, and the results must meet rigorous standards so that testers are unlikely to receive false negative or false positive results.

This section will cover the topic of DNA tests developed for medical purposes and how to choose a test that might be right for you. It provides the basics to get started and points you to specialists who can help you further.

Chapter 22:
DNA and your health

The Human Genome Project concluded around the turn of the twenty-first century, granting us a basic understanding of human DNA. The project revealed the order (or sequence) of DNA letters in a single individual's genome, but it did not explain what those DNA letters mean. The latter is now the primary work of genetics researchers today.

We know that most of the DNA letters tend to be ordered (or sequenced) in the same way for all people. The places where the DNA sequence can vary from the norm are called **variants**. Every day, new variants are discovered, which means some are well-understood and some are not.

> **Insider Tip:** Variants used to be called mutations, but now we know that some changes in the DNA are normal and not disease-causing. The community of genetics professionals has moved away from terminology like mutation that has a negative connotation.

Even with regular advances in genetics research, we are still in the early stages of understanding DNA as it relates to health and wellness. We know well the role of the *BRCA1* and *BRCA2* genes in some cases of cancers, for example, but DNA testing is still unveiling newly-discovered variants in these genes.

The more we test people's DNA, the more complicated we realize it is. Some new discoveries replace old understandings and re-write the rules. We dive into the world of DNA testing for health purposes in the next few chapters.

Chapter 23: Preparing for medical DNA testing

Your desire to do DNA testing might be driven by a need to find out hidden risks you carry or an explanation for your health problems. There are several different kinds of medical DNA tests that can help in these situations, each with strengths and weaknesses.

Before you get started

As you prepare for testing that might give medical or health information, here are questions to ask yourself:

- Am I ready for any type of result, whether positive, negative, or uncertain?

- Do I have a life insurance policy already in place?

- Do I know the uses and the limitations of the testing I want?

- Is this test medical-grade, or is it one that will need to be repeated for confirmation?

- Is this a test that requires family history to make full sense of the results?

- Is it possible to try to connect with biological relatives before making a final decision about testing?

- Have I checked with my insurance about the test coverage to find out my portion of the cost?

- When and how will I share the outcome of this testing with my children and other biological relatives?

The finer nuances

- ***Testing plus medical history together provide the best information***. The best understanding comes when family history, personal history, and results of high-quality, reliable genetic testing all come together; however, all that information may not always be available.

- **A DNA test cannot predict the future**. DNA is one part of a bigger picture when it comes to an understanding of what impacts our health. In many cases, a positive test does not necessarily mean you are destined for disease; alternatively, a negative test does not say you are in the clear.

- **Genetic testing cannot tell us about everything that runs in the family**. Genetic testing is not a replacement for family medical history since many conditions that run in the family are due to an interaction of multiple genes and environment.

- **What information you learn depends on the test you take**. Genetic tests are varied. Their reliability and usefulness hinge on the type of analysis done and the method used in decoding the results.

- **Sometimes a negative result is not genuinely negative**. A "negative" result might mean that the test focused on the wrong gene or skipped over the relevant location in the DNA; sometimes a negative result means a different test is needed for the disease-causing variant to be found.

- **Genetic risk is not fixed**. Our understanding of risk changes with time, due to collection of more information from research, family history, personal history, and new test results.

- **You can get shocking and upsetting information.** DNA tests can reveal information people thought they were prepared to find out but were not. Shock and trauma have happened to some who find out they have a higher risk for a devastating and currently untreatable condition, like Alzheimer disease, for example.

Different tests for different purposes

The following is a fictionalized story based on combining multiple, real stories. It introduces a few different types of tests and highlights their various uses. It also shows how the process of medical DNA testing is often done in steps, rather than all at once.

Kate and her husband Ryan met with Kate's gynecologist as they were preparing to start a family. The doctor had each of them take a saliva DNA test to screen for recessive conditions that could potentially affect their future children. Ryan did not know his ethnic background due to having been adopted as an infant, so the **certified genetic counselor** (see Chapter 26) they met with in the office recommended a specific type of test called an expanded carrier screen. Both Kate and Ryan received normal results.

Their infant son Aaron was born two years later with a cleft palate and some medical complications. Aaron's pediatrician referred him to a pediatric genetics clinic where a geneticist recommended testing Aaron's DNA using a combination of two approaches called karyotyping and chromosomal microarray analysis.

The results showed that Aaron had a portion of DNA missing in a region at the tip of one copy of chromosome 22. The other chromosome 22 appeared normal. The geneticist ordered parental testing, so both Kate and Ryan were tested but neither showed the same chromosome 22 deletion. This meant it most likely was a new genetic change that developed in Aaron.

Even with the reassurance that Aaron's genetic change was not something Ryan passed down to him, Ryan still wondered and worried about the lack of knowledge about his biological family's medical history. They spoke with the genetic counselor about what other options Ryan had for finding out about medical risks he might be passing on to his children. Although Ryan's insurance would not cover testing for him since he was healthy, he and Kate decided a proactive genetic screen held a lot of value for them. They used savings in their health spending account to cover the test costs (250 USD).

In this scenario, Kate and Ryan encountered multiple types of DNA testing for their family. Each DNA test was chosen with a clear goal in mind, and it was ordered with the support and guidance of a health care provider who could help Kate and Ryan understand the results when they came back.

Next, we cover some of the medical-grade DNA tests in more detail and point you to a specialist to pick the right test(s).

Chapter 24:
Medical-grade DNA testing

This section digs into the details of some of the different medical-grade DNA tests. Do not feel pressure to understand each option inside and out; instead, use this as a guide to begin learning.

> **WARNING:** DO NOT consider this section personal medical advice! We do not know your medical history or other pertinent information to make recommendations on specific tests for you. A certified genetic counselor or another medical genetics professional who reviews your individual goals and past medical history is best for that.

Carrier screening

This test is a well-established type of analysis that has been around for decades, commonly ordered on the expectant couple by a doctor during a pregnancy. **Carrier screening** looks for recessive gene variants that a person is unaware is being passed down through the family, as carriers have no symptoms or illness.

You might have heard of testing for cystic fibrosis, Tay-Sachs disease, or sickle cell anemia in the past. These are all examples of conditions tested on a carrier screen. Recessive conditions included in carrier screens typically have severe effects early in life or are milder conditions for which treatments and therapies are available.

In the past, carrier screening was ordered based on a person's ethnic background. Tay-Sachs screening was for Ashkenazi Jews and sickle cell screening for those of African descent, for example. Today, it is more common for everyone to receive a screen of many conditions before or during their childbearing years.

The large tests have been called pan-ethnic, universal, or **expanded carrier screening**. The change from focused testing based on ethnicity to expanded testing without concern for ethnicity is a positive change. Many people do not know their ethnic background, have been given wrong information by family, or have multiple ethnic backgrounds.

The conditions included on expanded carrier screens vary from one company to the next and one test to the next. Newer tests make it easier to test for multiple things all at once. Carrier screening is one of the most affordable and accessible medical-grade DNA test options. If insurance does not cover it (in many cases, it will), the out-of-pocket costs are similar to what you pay for an at-home DNA test.

Expanded carrier screening benefits those who are nearing or are in the childbearing years of life because the testing gives information for children's risks. It is one source of genetic information about yourself which does not require any involvement of biological family and benefits future generations.

Diagnostic genetic testing

If you are experiencing health issues or physical ailments that might be genetic in origin, **diagnostic testing** is the category of DNA testing a doctor might order. "Diagnostic" means the test is used to look for a diagnosis or root cause.

An oncologist might recommend testing *BRCA1, BRCA2,* and some other cancer-related genes for a woman who has developed ovarian cancer, for example. A neurologist might want to test for a neurodegenerative disorder called Huntington's disease if worrisome symptoms arise. These are two examples of diagnostic genetic tests ordered with a particular diagnosis in mind.

Insider Tip: Not all medical or health problems can be tied to a genetic cause or have a genetic test available yet. Fibromyalgia and other autoimmune conditions are an example of ones that have a genetic component but for which genetic testing is not currently available or of much help. Even with these types of challenges facing people with conditions that have a genetic component, medical professionals have an ever-growing list of tests to choose from.

The next scenario is based on an actual case to help explain how genetic testing that is *diagnostic* can be of help to an adoptee experiencing a medical issue.

Nell was a woman who developed breast cancer relatively young, in her early 40s. Her doctor asked if there was a family history, and Nell explained she was adopted as a child and did not know any recent family medical history. Her oncologist sent her to a certified genetic counselor to talk about the possible causes for her cancer and to understand more about her options for genetic testing.

The genetic counselor discussed that family history could help add to their understanding, but there are other ways to find out helpful information. He described to Nell a test called a cancer gene panel that would help look for some of the DNA variants seen in many cases of early-onset hereditary breast cancer. The test would look at approximately 20 genes, including the BRCA genes and more. Nell was relieved to find out she had options, and she decided to move forward with submitting a saliva sample for testing that day.

About a month later, Nell's genetic counselor called. He explained over the phone that her results showed a positive finding in a gene called *CHEK2*. It upset Nell and worried her at first, especially since she had never heard of the *CHEK2* gene before. The genetic counselor was reassuring. He helped Nell understand it was not her fault and her reaction to her result was normal. He gave information about what was known about the particular *CHEK2* finding she had and sent her information about a support group she could join to learn more.

Nell was relieved to learn that *CHEK2* increased her cancer risks but not as high as they might have been if her report had been BRCA positive instead. She asked her genetic counselor questions about testing her children, and he explained when testing is recommended in children and why. They discussed what monitoring for cancer would look like for others in the family until their genetic test results were known.

Nell began to think about searching for her birth family after her cancer diagnosis and DNA results. She realized that she now held information that could be important for biological relatives of hers who may not have any awareness of the increased genetic risk for cancer they might carry.

For adoptees who lack access to their full medical history, the right DNA test can provide powerful and useful information. If you have a medical condition or are having unexplained symptoms, a thoughtfully-chosen diagnostic test has the potential to save you from years wasted on a search for answers and can be helpful to you and your own children.

Diagnostic tests will grow in number over time. The scenario mentioned above describes only one of the types of DNA test that might be considered for you by your doctor or genetic counselor.

Pharmacogenomic testing

Pharmacogenomic testing, sometimes shortened to PGx testing, is a type of specialized DNA testing that looks at certain DNA variants in genes that influence an individual's reactions to certain medications. Many physician offices are starting to incorporate this testing into their care for patients. It can be helpful to all people, whether or not they know of a family history of adverse reaction to medications. Some options might become available on the at-home DNA testing market. Understand that they likely will be a partial analysis of the important variants rather than full. Medical-grade options still require an ordering healthcare provider, which makes access to them harder for some people.

> **Insider Tip:** The consumer DNA company 23andMe received approval to return pharmacogenomic results in 2018. Note there are significant limitations to 23andMe's testing. 23andMe only tests select markers spread out throughout the entire genome rather than looking at all of the relevant regions in each gene. Additionally, 23andMe and the FDA recommend that customers **repeat their testing in a medical-grade laboratory** before using the results for medical purposes. The 23andMe reports will offer many people a chance to receive genetic information that they otherwise might not have learned, but beware: some people have been falsely reassured or unnecessarily alarmed by their results.

Pharmacogenomic testing is most helpful to people who are prescribed certain types of medications. Statins (used for cholesterol management) and SSRIs (used for the treatment of major depression, anxiety, and other conditions) are two examples where a doctor's prescription might be modified based on your DNA results.

Like other categories of testing, the options for pharmacogenomic testing will grow with time. It is important to note that in some cases, the genes tested for pharmacogenomics purposes are often included in larger and more extensive tests, such as exome and genome tests (discussed later).

Proactive gene panel tests

You might not currently be experiencing medical issues but might have concerns about what conditions might be lurking in the future. A newer category of testing called **proactive screening** (also called preventative screening) has recently become available for this purpose. This development in the medical DNA testing market may be the best news yet for adoptees without access to their family history.

A proactive screen includes a set of well-understood genes. Genes are chosen because they are well-studied and known to be associated with cancer, cardiac disease, and some other conditions for which it helps to screen and monitor for ahead of time. Excluded from the gene list are ones for which there are no treatments or preventive steps at the moment (hereditary dementias, for example).

> **Insider Tip:** The list of genes included on these proactive tests is prepared carefully, to be able to give clear-cut answers for medical issues for which genetic causes can often be found. A proactive screen gives you a chance to gather extra information from medical-grade DNA testing without risking the psychological burden of getting back unclear or uncertain results.

Proactive screening is one way for adoptees to gain more information about their potential medical risks but without risking more uncertainty and getting back unclear results. Although diagnostic tests and proactive screens have a lot of overlap, there is one main difference: the reporting of a **VUS** if one is found. VUS stands for a variant of uncertain significance, and this is a gene change that might be cause for disease or might have no effect on our bodies. Without further study, it is hard to tell whether to be concerned or unconcerned about a VUS.

Insider Tip: You might hear VUS pronounced "vuss" or "voose," and both pronunciations are fine. A VUS will often get relabeled as pathogenic (harmful; potentially disease-causing) or benign (harmless) as researchers collect more data about other people who have that same change in their DNA.

A sample of one of these proactive screen reports (on testing ordered from the company Invitae) is shown next for educational purposes, to give you a sense of the type of information these medical-grade DNA tests can provide. A diagnostic report and a proactive screen would have a similar appearance. This image only shows a selection of a report that is nine pages long in full and contains more details about all the genes included on the test.

As of the publication date for this guide, only a few medical-grade DNA testing companies offer proactive genetic screening. Options will grow and change quickly which is typical for medical DNA tests.

Proactive screens are a newer approach to genetic testing, and standard medical recommendations have not caught up yet. Most health insurance companies do not yet recognize the medical value of DNA testing on healthy people. As a result, this testing will be an out-of-pocket expense for most people.

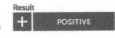
Screenshot showing a selection of a positive test report from a medical DNA test run by the medical-grade testing company Invitae. The actual report is nine pages in full.[5]

The cost of a proactive screen varies but can be expected to be in the range of 250-2,000 USD (2019 prices). Cost may place the testing out of reach for some people. For others, it will be a worthwhile investment for its potential to detect risks for a serious condition before its onset.

Some companies develop patient payment programs and cap the out-of-pocket expenses to make testing more affordable. Work with a certified genetic counselor to see what proactive tests are available (and at what cost) to you.

---

[5] Permission to review the full report and anonymously display the selection from the Invitae test report was granted to the authors by the individual tested.

Insider Tip: Not all genetics-trained professionals are familiar with or have worked with healthy people interested in proactive health screening. There is disagreement over the benefit of ordering extensive DNA testing on healthy individuals, and you will hear diverse opinions on the matter. The best approach may be to contact the companies offering proactive health screens and asking for a referral to a genetics specialist familiar with DNA testing on healthy people.

Over time, the number of genes on a proactive screen is expected to grow. Right now, more is not necessarily better because of the current limitations in understanding every possible result that can come back from DNA testing. The next section describes more extensive testing that covers greater regions of DNA and is becoming more commonplace.

Exome and genome testing

Exome and **genome tests** are the most extensive versions of testing currently available. The simplest explanation of the difference between an exome test and a genome test is how much of your DNA gets analyzed. Exome testing typically only focuses on the 1-2% of our DNA that is composed of genes. When we include the exome along with the other 98% of our DNA (regions outside of genes), we call that the genome.

The genome includes the DNA regions inside genes and the remaining DNA that connects genes as if they were beads on a string. The technology used for exome and genome testing is called sequencing, as opposed to genotyping, which is the prevalent technology for many at-home DNA tests and medical-grade options like some carrier screens.

> **Insider Tip:** There are a few different types of DNA sequencing tests, but as a group, sequencing tests analyze more genetic material than genotyping tests. *Sequencing* looks at DNA letters straight in a row for a long stretch of a gene, while *genotyping* plays a version of hopscotch through a gene, looking at a letter here and there.

Extensive DNA tests hold a lot of promise, especially for children and adults with rare diseases or with medical and developmental issues that have not yet been explained. Every day, new discoveries are making connections between genes and unexplained medical histories for many individuals. As a result, insurance coverage for extensive DNA testing continues to improve as the benefits become clearer.

Some individuals have begun to explore this more extensive testing even if they have no medical cause or reason for the testing. These individuals often want to know as much information as possible. You may count yourself in this group if you are a person who feels that knowledge is power and wants to be as well-informed as possible.

Any company that describes tests of the exome or genome as "whole exome or "whole genome" testing is bending the truth a bit. There are regions of the DNA that are more difficult to test, so all of these tests are missing some important regions in their analysis. DNA variations like pseudogenes (fake genes that mimic real ones) can obscure true results. Other types of DNA changes cannot be tested with the technology used for this type of DNA analysis, like the specific type of change in the DNA that leads to Fragile X syndrome, Huntington's disease, and many adult-onset neurologic disorders.

The availability of genome and exome testing depends on where you live. Some companies do not offer their testing internationally, or state laws place limits around the ordering of DNA testing within that state. In many situations, a healthcare provider's approval must be obtained either from a provider you know, a provider from a telemedicine network, or from one employed by the testing company itself. Research the details on a company's site and make sure you have found the one that fits your needs and is giving you information you seek.

Colin's Story

The next scenario is a combination of multiple real cases. It describes specific medical DNA tests and ways each is used to help adoptees to find information for themselves and their children.

Colin was a young boy adopted internationally. His parents knew of his special needs at the time of his adoption, which had been described in the medical records from his home country as autism and speech delay. His pediatrician referred him to the nearest pediatric genetics department as some cases of autism have an identifiable genetic cause. The clinical geneticist who saw Colin did a physical exam and collected all available history from Colin's parents. She came up with two specific tests to consider for Colin first: a microarray test and a gene panel test that focuses on over

2,300 genes known to be involved in some cases of autism and developmental delay.

The first test came back negative, so the geneticist ordered the autism gene panel test next. Colin's second test revealed a single genetic letter change in a gene called *SHANK3*, a gene associated with neurologic development. This gene had been implicated in many cases of autism in the past, and the geneticist felt this most likely explained Colin's neurological differences. If Colin's birth parents could ever provide samples, a focused DNA test of *SHANK3* could determine if the finding was a family variant rather than autism-associated. Testing birth parents was not an option at that time. Colin's parents and the doctor moved forward with an understanding that *SHANK3* was likely at play, but in the future as more information became available, their understanding of the cause for Colin's autism might change.

If Colin's second test had also been negative, the geneticist might have considered an exome or genome test next or might have suggested a return appointment in two or three years to discuss the newest test options.

Extensive tests like exome and genome analysis are more commonly done in people with undiagnosed diseases or medical issues. Some healthy individuals with the means to pay have extensive DNA testing as well, an approach some people refer to as healthy exome testing.

Expect to see this trend of more extensive testing—even on healthy people—continue into the future. It is a personal choice how much of your time, money, and emotional resources you invest into having DNA testing. But there is reason to believe that we will see the test costs drop, better information come from them, and easier access to professionals who can support you through testing.

Chapter 25: At-home DNA tests for health reasons

By this point, you will recognize that there are many varieties of DNA testing, some that are extensive and some that provide focused information. There are some options for testing that give back health information in which a provider does not have to be involved or is only minimally involved. We will look more at the benefits and limitations of these testing options next.

How to tell if an online DNA test is legitimate

Here is some advice on how to tell if a DNA test you find online and the company that sells it are legitimate:

- Check out the company website first. See if they identify the **people who run the company** by name, including their training and credentials.

- Take note of which **country** they are based in; some countries have lax laws about online business practices.

- The website should provide a **customer service hotline** or chat box for you to send in questions.

- The person you connect with over the phone should be familiar with new **terminology** you have come across in this section of the book, such as VUS, sequencing tests, and exome testing.

- The company should list at least one **genetic counselor** on their team, identified by name and with verifiable credentials. Testing companies that employ genetic counselors place value on clear communication and support for DNA test customers who have questions.

- Are they selling a different product, such as vitamin supplements or a sauna, and using DNA testing to encourage you to buy their other product?

Health + Ancestry reports

23andMe and MyHeritage are the better-known at-home DNA testing companies providing medical genetics reports. They differ in the way the tests are activated online and how medical providers (like doctors and genetic counselors) are involved in the process. Whether using 23andMe or MyHeritage, you must order or upgrade to the Health + Ancestry testing option to get medical reports which costs more than their ancestry-only test.

In the U.S., 23andMe has FDA approval to provide their reports without having an ordering healthcare provider involved. MyHeritage has partnered with a medical service to review information you provide before activating your kit. MyHeritage has genetic counselors involved before and after the testing is done; 23andMe does not.

Other lesser-known companies, like Color Genomics and Helix, have a similar set-up to MyHeritage with ordering providers involved at one or more steps in the process. Each of these companies has a different business model, different reports, and will create a different experience for you.

DNA tests vary around the globe, and you might not have access to all of them based on where you live. The next steps to take after you receive results are to confirm any positive results by taking a second (clinical-grade) DNA test before taking any action. 23andMe provides you a link to a search tool for locating a genetic counselor, and MyHeritage established a process for getting you connected to one.

Both 23andMe and MyHeritage's Health + Ancestry test provides a set of carrier screen reports, ones with health risk data, and at least one **polygenic** risk report. Polygenic refers to the fact that many variants (possibly hundreds or thousands) in the DNA are involved in the genetics of a condition rather than just one or a few. 23andMe's FDA approval extends to pharmacogenomics reports as well. It is not clear at this time whether MyHeritage will offer these types of reports in the future.

A report from these companies might tell you if you are a carrier of a few select variants seen in some cases of a genetic condition. The testing does not sequence the entire gene involved. Your report may list a finding that elevates your chance for Alzheimer's disease or age-related macular degeneration, but other factors are often stronger predictors of these conditions than the DNA variants. None of these reports are diagnosing you with disease, and none predict whether you actually will develop that condition during your life.

Each company reports limitations, but you might need to hunt for them and make an effort to understand what they mean. Here is an example of how 23andMe. This "Keep in mind" section is provided near the bottom and points out that: points out that:

- the test does not diagnose disease
- other factors (age, weight, ethnicity, etc.) are at play
- that they do not test for all disease variants
- the report is based on research findings that have not been confirmed with repeated testing that is clinical grade

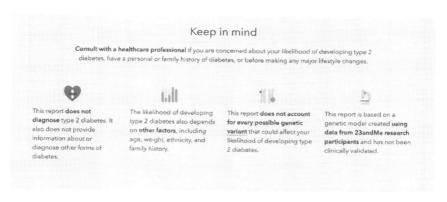

Keep in mind

Consult with a healthcare professional if you are concerned about your likelihood of developing type 2 diabetes, have a personal or family history of diabetes, or before making any major lifestyle changes.

This report does not diagnose type 2 diabetes. It also does not provide information about or diagnose other forms of diabetes.

The likelihood of developing type 2 diabetes also depends on other factors, including age, weight, ethnicity, and family history.

This report does not account for every possible genetic variant that could affect your likelihood of developing type 2 diabetes.

This report is based on a genetic model created using data from 23andMe research participants and has not been clinically validated.

If medical DNA testing were a multi-course meal, the DNA health reports offered by 23andMe and MyHeritage can be thought of as the appetizer. It is easy to become falsely alarmed or falsely reassured unless you take the time to understand the limits of each report. Make sure to read through the scientific details to understand everything the testing report can and cannot tell you. A genetic counselor can be a partner for this, especially if you have a lot of questions that arise as you read through the findings.

> **Insider Tip:** At-home BRCA testing is of limited use for most people. You can have a normal BRCA report from 23andMe or MyHeritage and still have a cancer-causing variant in the *BRCA1* or *BRCA2* gene that could predispose you to developing cancer. Or, you might have a variant in a cancer gene not tested at all. 23andMe only reports on **three** out of the thousands known to exist in the BRCA genes. These three variants are found in some people who have Ashkenazi Jewish background. MyHeritage looks at additional BRCA variants, but neither company sequences the BRCA genes.

At-home DNA testing for medical reasons will continue to grow in the future. They can be an important way for you to learn about a few conditions with known genetic causes and to learn about how genes are one factor influencing disease. If you test with an at-home company like 23andMe or MyHeritage, think of your results as the start of your journey into seeking out medical information, not as the end.

Using raw data files for health information

23andMe, MyHeritage, and other at-home DNA companies that have an ancestry focus use a genetic technology called genotyping. These companies often allow you to download raw data files of your genotyped DNA markers.

Genotype files include a small portion of your DNA, not a read-out of your complete DNA sequence. The DNA locations (sometimes referred to as markers or SNPs) included in a raw data file differ from one company to the next. Each company can specify which locations they want to include or remove from the analysis. What appears on a third party report produced from the raw data file also differs depending on the company's file you use and whether the third party analysis filters out and reports it.

> **Insider Tip:** Understand that raw data is just that – *raw*. These files do not include the complete sequence of your genome, and they contain errors which are impossible for individual users to spot. If you choose to run your raw data file through a health analysis tool, think of your results as a head start and not the end point. There are caveats to all third-party health tools that scan a raw data file, and your DNA testing should be repeated in a medical-grade testing laboratory.

Promethease and other third-party health tools

Promethease, Sequencing.com, and Xcode Life are a few of the more common third-party tools discussed in DNA and genealogy groups. These are some options for seeking potential health information from a DNA raw data file. More options will likely become available with time.

These websites offer analysis to paying customers using raw data files produced elsewhere, typically an at-home DNA testing company. Third-party tools rely on proprietary filtering techniques to dig deeper into a raw data file and report these to you.

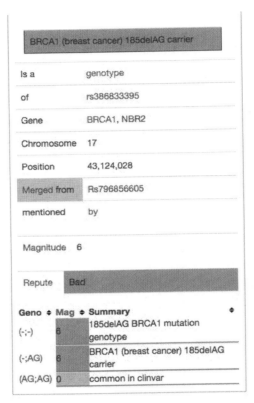

Screenshot of one of the hundreds or thousands of entries that can appear in a Promethease report. The report links to this display of information on a free wiki site called SNPedia.

You will see Promethease mentioned more often in online genealogy groups, likely to due to greater familiarity with this particular tool, so we will explore this one in a little more detail.

Promethease relies on an online encyclopedia of medical genetics research called SNPedia to filter the raw data file and report on findings present. The database of research in

SNPedia is always growing, which means the report changes over time. What is present on your report depends on the company's raw data file you provide.

> **Insider Tip:** Your third-party health report will change over time even though your DNA stays the same. This is because DNA markers that are tested often change from one version of a company's test to the next. Also, genetics research is always changing, and some DNA variants initially thought to be harmful turn out to be benign (and vice versa).

Many people have reported that a Promethease report can be overwhelming at first glance, and it is not intuitive how to use it to sort through and find useful information. The other tools may provide reports that are more visually appealing. No matter how the information is displayed, remember that all third-party analyses that rely on raw data files from at-home tests have various caveats and limitations (highlighted earlier).

Brianne has developed an online video and some tips on her blog to help you get started if you decide to use raw data and third-party tools like Promethease. The developers of Promethease have also helped their users by developing a few online videos, providing support pages on SNPedia, and identifying and reporting common false positive findings to testers, which they label with the term "miscall."

Miscall for 23andMe customers; otherwise: Unaffected carrier of a Smith-Lemli-Opitz syndrome mutation	
Is a	genotype
of	rs80338859
Gene	DHCR7
Chromosome	11

Screenshot showing how a possible miscall (false positive) is reported when it is discovered by SNPedia/Promethease

Promethease's developers maintain a list of certified genetic counselors who can help you understand your report. Search the SNPedia website for information on how to find a genetic counselor who can help, or do an Internet search to find those who list "direct-to-consumer testing" as a specialty.

Genetic tests for nutrition and exercise

You might be interested in DNA testing in all its forms, ranging from tests that help with family searching to those that provide medical or nutritional information. You are likely to come across a website or person at some point that promises to guide you to the right diet, vitamins, or exercise routines based on your DNA.

This is a controversial area in DNA testing. There is no consensus that the science is solid behind most of the claims. Genes and variants in genes have an impact on cell metabolism, but this does not automatically mean that the recommendations to take certain supplements, follow certain diets, or detoxify your body are backed by evidence. Yet you will see individual providers (and even some of the big at-home DNA testing companies) selling test reports that claim to be customized for you.

Rather than telling you what and who to believe on this topic, we will equip you with information to help you start to assess the claims yourself. First, understand that recommendations are for the most part being based on analysis of raw data files produced by genotyping. Recall from earlier sections that raw data files change over time and have undetectable errors. Genotyping (the technology which most commonly produces the raw data files) only tests a small number of the DNA letters (the markers or SNPs) from your entire genome.

Specialized supplements marketed to promote health have not been studied in **placebo-controlled studies**. These are the types of studies which pit placebo pills taken by one group of people against a pill with active ingredients to see if the active ingredients have any effect. Because dietary supplements are not treated the way medications and other therapies are, the evidence is lacking at this time that supplements--including special folate supplements recommended based on *MTHFR* gene findings--have the effects on your body that those who sell them claim they do.

The studies being cited to support claims about genetically-determined supplements tend to be from a category called **genome-wide association studies** (GWAS). These studies of large groups of people look for "hotspots" in the genome that might be associated with diseases or traits. Follow-up studies must be done after GWAS to determine if the association truly exists and if so, why. These follow-up studies are lacking for most of the claims being made about genetically-determined supplement and dietary changes. From a desire to help people feel better and optimize their health based on any available evidence, those who recommend DNA testing for this purpose might not realize that the science they are citing for support has skipped over this important follow-up step.

GWAS study findings can be applied to groups of people but not individuals within that group. In other words, it might be true that other people with similar DNA results to yours respond to a supplement, diet, or exercise routine in a certain way; because you are genetically unique and have a different combination of genetic variants, it does not mean you will respond the same way others in the group do.

The dietary supplements industry is generally unregulated around the globe, so regulating bodies like the U.S. FDA do not oversee companies operating in this area. It is the wild west of DNA testing, and almost anyone can claim what they want to about supplements, diet, and exercise based on DNA as long as they provide in fine print that it is for educational purposes and not intended to be medical advice.

All this said, it is also true that some people do have nutritional deficiencies and metabolic disorders that call for modified diets and therapies. Many of the conditions automatically tested for in newborn babies using a blood draw from a heel stick soon after birth are genetically-determined metabolic conditions, for example. Because of this gray zone in the areas of metabolic and nutrition genetics, it makes it hard to know when you are being given reliable information.

> **Insider Tip:** There is no easy way to evaluate people promoting nutrigenomics to determine if they understand the difference between GWAS studies and placebo-controlled studies or whether they grasp the challenge of using DNA results on groups of people to make custom recommendations for you. Your best approach at this point in time is to work with someone with advanced degrees in both nutrition and human genetics who does not also attempt to sell you supplements or otherwise benefit from you buying a product or service based on a DNA report.

Chapter 26:
Working with a Certified Genetic Counselor

What is a Certified Genetic Counselor?

Certified Genetic Counselors are masters-trained professionals with experience in both genetics and counseling. They guide and support patients, clients, and families who are making decisions around DNA testing. They also assist those with questions after having the testing. Most genetic counselors work in the health/medical setting, many of them as part of a medical clinic or telemedicine network (services provided over the phone or Internet).

Just as there are many different types of doctors, there are many different types of genetic counselors. Some are highly specialized in a certain medical area or help with behind-the-scenes tasks at DNA testing companies. Some have roles in the education of students, other providers, and the general public. Some work with rare disease patient groups or in industry.

A *clinical* genetic counselor – one who works directly with patients or clients – is the best fit as a personal guide. They help you figure out which (if any) testing is right for you. More clinical genetic counselors are becoming well-versed in addressing common issues that arise with at-home testing, genome and exome testing, pharmacogenomics, and other areas of special interest to adoptees.

There are many reasons to consider working with a genetic counselor. They assist with:

- selecting the right test for you
- finding out the after-insurance costs to you for medical-grade testing

- locating a lab that will repeat findings from an at-home DNA test for confirmation

- making sure your rights and wishes are respected

- handling the ordering of a test and returning the final results to you

- explaining the usual recommendations after a positive or negative result

- helping you navigate challenging discussions with your family

- assisting and advising other medical professionals involved in your care or your child's care

Insider Tip: If you are seeking a medical DNA test, there are benefits to involving a medical genetics professional. Certified genetic counselors are important partners when fitting DNA tests results into your care. They match the best test to your needs and work to cut down on the unnecessary panic, false reassurance, and test misinterpretations that often occur after DNA testing. Genetics nurses and medical geneticists are also helpful in many situations and might be available to assist you as well.

Concerns about costs

Some people are concerned about the price of medical-grade DNA tests or genetic counseling services. In many situations, you may qualify for fully-covered testing and genetic counseling if your doctor advises it or if you meet insurance criteria.

Some genetic testing companies have also designed programs to help make testing affordable to those who have to contribute personally to cover a test or the services around it. These patient-friendly companies have developed patient payment plans, financial assistance programs, and benefits investigation (BI) services to check on test coverage with your insurance company for you. Some employ genetic counselors in-house so that if you call with questions, someone on the other end of line will be able to answer them.

You might consider using contributions to a health spending account or apply your insurance deductible towards test coverage and genetic counseling costs. Using different approaches to financing a test can limit the impact on your family's budget and make services and testing more affordable.

> **Insider Tip:** Before assuming that medical-grade DNA testing is out of reach for you, set up an appointment (online or in person) with a certified genetic counselor to find out the various options you have. You might be surprised to learn that some medical-grade tests are available at the same cost as one or a few at-home tests.

Concerns about genetic discrimination

Concerns about genetic discrimination are often raised by people interested in having DNA testing. U.S. and Canada residents are guaranteed some legal protection from discrimination based on genetic information. A certified genetic counselor can make sure you have an accurate understanding of the actual risks of having a DNA test.

The **Genetic Information Non-discrimination Act** (GINA) is a U.S. federal law passed in 2008. Canada passed a similar law, Genetic Non-Discrimination Act or GNA, in 2017. These laws offer protection against certain situations of employment and insurance discrimination.

GINA excludes certain types of insurance such as life insurance and long-term disability plans, so consider looking into insurance options *before* you have any DNA testing.

Inaccurate reporting of the testing you have had or lying on an application can invalidate the policy.

Many DNA tests that are medical-grade can be of a cost similar to those in the at-home test market. Some people have decided to pay out of pocket for testing so that their insurance company is not involved. This can also cut down on the potential opportunities for discrimination.

Weigh the benefits of having reliable information from a medical-grade DNA test against the potential harms, and make the best decision that you can. There is no single decision that is right for every person or family. See the links in the resources section to find more information about GINA and GNA protections for U.S. and Canadian residents.

Locating a Certified Genetic Counselor

Although not every experience with a genetic counselor will be the same, working with one can save you time, frustration, and money. Barriers to access have been reduced in recent years, due to developments like telemedicine services.

Here are some ideas on how to find a specialist you can talk to about genetic testing:

- Search online to find a genetic counselor near you, and contact them to see if they accept self-referred patients (see resources section for search tools).

- Ask your primary care physician to refer you to a genetic counselor or genetics clinic in your healthcare system or area.

- Search on your insurance provider's website for in-network providers.

- Search for a nationwide genetics network, like Genome Medical or Grey Genetics, and refer yourself for a virtual genetic counseling session.

- Seek out online videos and education created by genetic counselors and other medical specialists.

- Reach out to work with Brianne through her private practice, Watershed DNA (*some state residency restrictions apply*).

Many other specialists in other areas like maternal-fetal medicine, oncology, cardiology, and neurology have also undergone extra training in medical genetics or work closely with genetics-trained colleagues. These teams can be a great resource for you in your search for information from a medical DNA test.

You may find that some clinicians have more experience working with adoptees than others, generally based on years in practice and areas of specialization. We wrote about adoption-competent counselors earlier on in the book. There is no easy way to identify adoption-competent genetics specialists at this time.

The information you learn from a medical DNA test can have life-long benefits for you and future generations. Seek out advice from those familiar with all of your different options, and consider the time, effort, and expense spent on medical-grade testing as a worthwhile investment for you and your family.

Chapter 27: Accessing family health history

Information from a DNA test can be one way to gather information, but a family medical history can be a valuable source of information as well. If you make contact with biological family, an interest in medical history might already be at the top of your list. It need not be seen as rude or morbid if medical history is one of the first things you ask about. Talking about death and illness can feel uncomfortable (especially with someone who might be a stranger to you) but remind yourself this information is important.

Questions to ask

Here are a few things to ask biological family about health:

- What were the ages and causes of death of my close family members?

- Do you have any details about the type or age of onset for anyone in the family who had cancer?

- Regarding cardiovascular health, did anyone die suddenly or unexpectedly as a young person? Any infant deaths? Chronic issues like high cholesterol or high blood pressure?

- Did anyone develop dementia early in life, have neurological issues, or have medical issues during their childhood?

- Is the family part of an isolated population (Amish, ethnic Jewish, etc.) or have any situations of intermarriage in recent generations?

You may wish to send a family history form you get from your doctor or one you find online. Ask biological family if they would be willing to help you fill it out to the best of their knowledge. Offer to share your medical history with them as well, if you feel comfortable doing that. Sharing medical history is a two-way street, and what you can offer might help your biological relatives as well.

Some people have not been able to get helpful information from a close biological relative like a parent or sibling but have gathered this from a cousin who knows about the family. Some have collected additional information about causes of death listed in the public family trees or from other places, such as death certificates, obituaries, and online memorials.

Many people who participate in DNA testing for genealogical purposes are willing to help if you ask. Gather this information for the benefit of yourself and future generations, even if you must repeatedly ask. Seek out answers from someone else in the family if the first person closes the door on a medical history discussion.

Getting health information from your adoption records

Consider the documents search advice in Chapter 2 to investigate your options and determine whether health information is something you might be able to request from your adoption records. Even if you were adopted in a closed-records state, you may have a legal right to this information. Consider this next case of a gentleman named Bill with whom Brianne worked.

Bill was a healthy 65-year old who was adopted at birth in a closed adoption. He had been happily married to his wife for decades, and they had multiple children and many grandchildren. Bill said he had always felt guilty that he was unable to provide his own family with any medical history besides his own. He learned that if he petitioned the court, he might be able to gain access to health history information and did so successfully.

Bill received a health summary from his file and learned that aside from a few relatives with elevated blood pressure and history of cigarette smoking, his biological family members appeared to have been generally healthy and long-lived. Months later, Bill identified biological family using DNA testing. After making contact with his biological mother and siblings, he was able to obtain new medical information that had developed in the decades since the brief history was placed in his file.

Insider Tip: Health information is considered non-ID information, meaning you often have rights to access these records even if your adoption records are sealed. You may need to apply for the medical information in writing. Check out the website for the agency or department in charge of adoption records in your state to find out the specifics that apply to your situation.

Chapter 28:
Special issues for adoptive parents and minors

Parents children who were adopted and are still minors have reached out to ask about using DNA testing to help their children. DNA testing is clearly on the radar for many of these families, for various reasons.

The focus of this section is on topics relevant to parents of adopted children who are under the age of 18, but these points can apply to other families as well.

Because of societal shifts and changing legislation, parents adopting children today are faced with a different world than adoptive parents of past decades and generations. Adoptive parents of the current time are often thinking about and preparing for a discussion about biological family and DNA testing long before an adopted child broaches the topic. For all adoptive parents, it is important to have a basic understanding of DNA tests and what they can and cannot reveal.

There are four components to DNA testing that adoptive parents should be aware of. Most of these come from tests available on the at-home DNA test market, but the third bullet point straddles both the medical and at-home testing spheres. Current DNA options that are most important to be aware of are:

- Ethnic background estimation (ethnicity pie chart)
- Genetic family matching (DNA Relatives, Family Finder, etc.)
- Health/medical-related reports (various types that differ in the depth and quality of data provided)
- Raw data (the unprocessed computerized file of DNA markers, typically from an at-home DNA test)

Adoptive parents and their adopted children may feel differently about the importance of DNA to determining who is or is not family. Not every adopted person feels the same about the significance of DNA as part of their identity. Not every adoptee decides to pursue DNA testing or a relationship with birth family. Support your child's uniqueness and stay open and receptive to their thoughts about DNA testing.

When an adopted child asks about DNA testing

A person's interest or lack of interest in DNA testing is not a reflection on the parenting they receive. One adoptee posted the following about the diversity of adoptee perspectives and experiences on a social network to which we authors belong:

"There is no normal. We each have our own story. We all have different needs and questions."

The right time to discuss DNA and to order DNA testing varies from one person to the next. Sometimes childhood is the right time to order a test, and sometimes waiting until adulthood is better.

Insider Tip: Information on ethnicity can be important for some people as they form an identity, especially in late childhood or early adolescence and if their ethnicity differs from that of their adoptive family. In fact, DNA testing to find out ethnic background is often the information adopted individuals express interest in first.

Be willing to listen and support your child in their decisions about DNA testing. You may wish to set a time frame or a minimum age for testing for your family. Be willing to flex on the issue if your child has a different perspective and does not want to wait.

Special consideration about family matching databases

You do not have to opt in to the family matching feature to order DNA testing on your adopted child. That aspect of DNA testing can be considered later and can have importance later in life. For example, many adopted individuals say they would have felt differently about who they could date and marry if they had reassurance they were not going to accidentally meet up with a biological relative.

The concern of accidentally running into biological family and not knowing it is a legitimate one. It is possible that due to a closed adoption or a situation in which the paternity of a child is unknown or has been reported falsely, siblings or cousins may inadvertently date. It is rare but is known to have happened. This is a point to keep in mind as your child gets older.

Obtaining health information for your child

Trying to obtain family medical history on an ongoing basis from biological family is ideal, but different challenges involved in adoption might make this difficult. Medical professionals understand the value of a family history and often are left wondering how to fill in the gap in those situations when history is not available. This can be frustrating for everyone – the parents, the child, and the healthcare provider.

The National Society of Genetic Counselors developed the following position statement about collecting health information for children in the process of being adopted to emphasize the importance of this information:

> **Genetic Testing of Children in the Adoption Process**: The National Society of Genetic Counselors (NSGC) supports collecting available health information (including medical, genetic, and family history) for children entering the adoption process. As with any child, concerns that arise about a genetic condition should be relayed to a clinical genetics specialist to determine if genetic testing is appropriate. Decisions to genetically test a child during the adoption process should be made based on the child's current medical needs and should not be used solely to decide whether to adopt the child. Prior to finalizing the adoption, NSGC recommends that the adoption agency or child's representative confirm the biological and adoptive parents' preferences for re-contact regarding genetic test results or medically significant family history. (*NSGC 2018; www.nsgc.org*)

The topics raised by this statement involve situations that are complex and nuanced. Medical needs are a deciding factor for some families to move forward with an adoption for a child, and it is challenging to succinctly address all various questions DNA testing can raise. Chapter 2 covers records searches for international/intercountry adoptions in more detail, and Chapters 24-26 cover medical topics for adoptees. We recommend connecting with adoptive parent groups for discussions on specific topics that go beyond these two areas.

Adopted children with health concerns

For families whose adopted child is having health issues or has other special needs of unclear cause, consider asking your pediatrician to refer you to a medical genetics clinic. You might search for a pediatric genetic counselor in your area or a genetics clinic that has special adoption clinics where they are prepared to address the unique needs of adopted children. The resources section includes information on a search tool for locating a genetic counselor. An adoptive parents group might be another resource.

At-home testing has major gaps in DNA coverage at this time, and it does not meet the level of completeness recommended for seeking out a medical diagnosis or making medical predictions. The prior chapters cover these topics in greater depth.

Seeking out information for hidden health risks

Healthy individuals often approach DNA testing without any particular medical concern in mind. They may instead want to know about potential hidden risks. Consider looking into "proactive" health tests covered previously. Many professionals who work with children and DNA testing will recommend that you allow your child to decide for themselves when and whether they have a medical DNA test once they reach adulthood, if the information that can come from testing will not have any immediate impact on them or their medical care. Some tests can be ordered on healthy children, and these options expand and change every year.

There are some outcomes to consider before moving forward with DNA testing. There is no legal protection against discrimination for life and long-term disability insurance, for example, and anti-discrimination laws like GINA and GNA do not cover all situations. The benefits and the risks of doing DNA testing on a healthy person are varied, whether that person is an adult or a child.

Using raw data from an at-home DNA test

Be careful of websites and online tools you find that encourage you to submit a raw data file from another company's testing for more health/medical information. There are many limitations to these tools—and risks for false positives and negatives (plus false reassurance) when using raw data files. When it involves DNA testing on you, it is one thing. But this is nothing to take lightly when thinking about health and medical information for a child.

There are many different companies that offer at-home DNA testing and medical-grade testing, and the options are growing. To pick a test that meets the needs of your child, look for a medical genetics professional to work with who has a solid understanding of the different types of tests and the rights you turn over to the company when you submit a DNA sample to a testing company.

Final thoughts on DNA testing and adopted children

There is a lot to be gained from considering DNA testing for your adopted child. Be willing to have open conversations and consider your child's perspective. Even young children can have insight into the benefits that can come from looking into their DNA.

As your child nears the age of adulthood, it will be important to think about transitioning DNA accounts, login credentials, and DNA reports to them.

Part 4 - Takeaway Points

- Different technologies are used to detect different genetic differences with a medical impact.

- Medical tests regularly uncover new genetic variants that we do not yet understand.

- Five types of tests adoptees might consider pursuing are: expanded carrier screening, pharmacogenomic testing, diagnostic testing, proactive genetic screening, and/or extensive screening of the exome or genome.

- DNA tests developed for at-home purposes do not analyze all the markers related to medical issues and predispositions.

- Raw data files from consumer ancestry tests have limitations, like undetected errors, that make them of limited use for medical purposes.

- Incomplete knowledge about DNA variants means we are dealing with uncertain findings on a regular basis.

- A few at-home test companies like 23andMe and MyHeritage provide some medical DNA reports; check the fine print for their recommendations about repeat testing in a clinical lab before using it for medical purposes.

- Certified genetic counselors and other genetics-trained specialists can help you pick a DNA test that fits your goals and help you understand the results.

- The dropping costs of DNA testing are making medical-grade tests more accessible, whether insurance coverage is involved.

- Adoptive parents have special considerations to take into account when ordering DNA testing on minors, but there are potential benefits to testing.

Epilogue:
Bringing it all together

In previous chapters, we cover a lot of ground. We mention the various parties involved in helping with a search, like search angels, professional genetic genealogists, and confidential intermediaries. We reviewed the different uses of information that come from testing the autosomal DNA, the Y and X chromosomes, and mitochondrial DNA. The medical section at the end covers a range of different topics, including medical-grade tests and various at-home options.

There is a lot of information you can gather ahead of time, and some you will not know you need until you get started down the path. We hope this book serves as a useful guide for your journey, no matter which sections apply in your situation.

If you find yourself stuck after you get started, try these things:

- Test at another company.

- Check to see if any of your matches have updated their information (last names, family trees, etc.).

- Upload your raw data file to any remaining matching databases.

- Try more advanced work with your match data (triangulation, segment data work, color clustering, automatic clustering, phasing, etc.).

- Share your frustrations with others who have also searched, and see if they have tips for you.

- Ask for help from others (family or friends with interest in DNA searching, search angel groups, Facebook groups for DNA family searches, paid professionals, etc.).

- Make a mirror tree at Ancestry.com only as a last resort. (Caution! Make this tree private and non-searchable. You may want to let an experienced searcher do this for you.)

If you are still stuck, a little passage of time might give your biological family members more time to DNA test and appear as matches to you in your list. You might wish to check in every few months to see if new tools to analyze DNA matches have been developed, or if any new testing companies or databases have appeared.

We asked one adoptee named Karen when she knew her search was complete, after she had already connected with both sides of her birth family and had DNA testing for health reasons. "That's a great question," she answered. "I'm not sure if it is complete. There are still questions I have every time I think about history."

Perhaps like Karen, finding answers will be the start of a new set of questions for you. Following this epilogue is a list of resources that you can turn to. These extra supports include books, online groups, and websites.

Making the effort to learn about your biological family is more than just tracking down the basic facts of your existence. Discoveries we make about biological origins inform our personal identities and influence who we are and how we feel about our place in the world.

This journey for information might be one of the most significant life milestones for you. What happens might bring a sense of closure, happiness, or satisfaction. It might also stir up buried emotions and lead you to re-experience traumas from your past. We hope that if this happens to you, you will let those around you know what you are going through, and reach out to a counseling professional.

If your search leads you to discover something shocking and unexpected, such as information that you were conceived during a sexual assault or have high ROH, there is specialized support for you. If you cannot find your way to this support on your own, please reach out to us (the authors) directly, and we will help connect you.

We wish the very best to you in your search for information. A book cannot cover all the potential aspects of the journey for you, but we hope this one has served as a source of encouragement for you to get started and that you return to it for continued support and information in the future.

If you have found parts of the book to be especially helpful or that could use improvement in future editions, please reach out and let us know. Both of us authors would love to hear from you.

- Brianne and Shannon

Appendix of Resources

Books

- Aulicino, Emily D. Genetic Genealogy: The Basics and Beyond. AuthorHouse, 2013.

- Bettinger, Blaine The Family Tree Guide to DNA Testing and Genetic Genealogy. Cincinnati, OH: Family Tree Books, 2016.

- Dowell, David R. Nextgen Genealogy: The DNA Connection. Santa Barbara, California: Libraries Unlimited, 2015.

- Kennett, Debbie. DNA and Social Networking: A Guide to Genealogy in the Twenty-first Century. Stroud: History Press, 2011.

- Redmonds, George, and Turi King. Surnames, DNA, and Family History. Oxford: Oxford University Press, 2011.

- Smolenyak, Megan, and Ann Turner. Trace Your Roots with DNA: Using Genetic Tests to Explore Your Family Tree. Emmaus, PA: Rodale, 2004.

- Weinberg, Tamar The Adoptee's Guide to DNA Testing. Cincinnati, OH: Family Tree Books, 2018.

- Wells, Spencer. Deep Ancestry: Inside the Genographic Project. Washington, D.C.: National Geographic, 2006.

Genealogy and DNA blogs

- Bettinger, Blaine, **The Genetic Genealogist**
  https://thegeneticgenealogist.com

- Christmas, Shannon, **Through the Trees**
  https://www.Throughthetreesblog.tumblr.com

- Combs-Bennett, Shannon, **TNT Family History**
  https://tntfamilyhistory.blogspot.com

- Cooper, Kitty, **Kitty Cooper's Blog**
  https://blog.kittycooper.com/

- Dowell, David, **Dr D Digs Up Ancestors**
  https://blog.ddowell.com

- Estes, Roberta, **DNAeXplained – Genetic Genealogy**
  https://dna-explained.com

- **Family Tree Magazine** (DNA articles, news, and advice)
  https://www.familytreemagazine.com/articles/news-blogs/

- Hill, Richard, **DNA Testing Adviser**
  https://www.dna-testing-adviser.com

- Kennett, Debbie, **Cruwys News**
  https://www.Cruwys.blogspot.com

- Kirkpatrick, Brianne, **Watershed DNA**
  https://www.watersheddna.com/blog-and-news/

- Larkin, Leah, **The DNA Geek**
  https://www.thednageek.com

- Moore, CeCe, **Your Genetic Genealogist**
  https://www.yourgeneticgenealogist.com

- Russell, Judy, **The Legal Genealogist**
  https://www.legalgenealogist.com/

- Southard, Diahan, **Your DNA Guide**
  https://www.yourdnaguide.com

- Wayne Debbie Parker, **Deb's Delvings**
  https://www.debsdelvings.blogpost.com

Facebook groups

- **Adoption and DNA**
  https://www.facebook.com/adoptiondna/
- **Adoption Search and Reunion**
  https://www.facebook.com/groups/57164728955/
- **DNAadoption**
  https://www.facebook.com/DNAAdoption/
- **DNA Detectives**
  https://www.facebook.com/groups/DNADetectives/
- **GEDmatch User Group**
  https://www.facebook.com/groups/gedmatchuser/
- **Genetic Genealogy Tips and Techniques**
  https://www.facebook.com/groups/geneticgenealogytips
  andtechniques/
- **Revelations Opening Up About Family for Adoptees and Adopters**
  https://www.facebook.com/adoptioncommunity/
- **Search Squad**
  https://www.facebook.com/groups/searchelpers/
- **Visual Phasing**
  https://www.facebook.com/groups/visualphasing/

Podcasts

- **AdopteesOn**
  http://www.adopteeson.com/
- **Extreme Genes**
  https://extremegenes.com/
- **Genealogy Happy Hour**
  https://genealogyhappyhour.com/
- **The Genealogy Guys Podcast**
  http://www.genealogyguys.com/

Websites for adoption-specific topics

- **DNA Adoption – Reference Documentation**
  http://dnaadoption.com/index.php?page=reference-documentation

Websites for common ancestry testing companies

- **23andMe**
  https://www.23andme.com

- **Ancestry**
  https://www.ancestry.com/dna/

- **Family Tree DNA**
  https://www.familytreedna.com

- **Living DNA**
  https://livingdna.com

- **MyHeritage**
  https://www.myheritage.com/dna

- **National Geographic**
  https://genographic.nationalgeographic.com

Websites for genealogy

- **Cyndi's List – Surnames – DNA**
  https://www.cyndislist.com/surnames/dna/

- **Family Tree DNA (FTDNA) Projects**
  https://www.familytreedna.com/projects.aspx?

- **Genetic Genealogy Standards Committee**
  https://www.geneticgenealogystandards.com

- **International Society of Genetic Genealogy**
  https://isogg.org

- **The Surname Society**
  https://surname-society.org/

Websites for medical and counseling support

- **AdopteesOn**
  https://www.adopteeson.com/listen/chooseatherapist

- **Genetic Counselors**
  https://www.findageneticcounselor.com/ (search tool for U.S. genetic counselors)

  https://www.abgc.net/about-genetic-counseling/find-a-certified-counselor.aspx/ (search tool for CGCs)

  https://www.cagc-accg.ca (search tool for Canadian genetic counselors)

- **Psychology Today**
  https://www.psychologytoday.com/ (search tool for therapists/licensed professional counselors)

- **Genetics Home Reference – NIH**
  https://ghr.nlm.nih.gov/
  (a reliable source of information about medical genetic conditions)

- **Genetic Discrimination Information** (quick guides for understanding genetic discrimination protections in the U.S. and Canada)

  http://www.ginahelp.org/GINA_you.pdf (U.S.)

  https://www.cagc-accg.ca/doc/revised%20GNA%20fact%20sheet%20-%20Jun%2028%202018.pdf (Canada)

Additional genetics websites and third-party tools

- **Promethease**
  https://promethease.com/

- **Sequencing.com**
  https://sequencing.com/

- **Xcode Life**
  https://www.xcode.life/

- **DNAGedcom**
  https://www.dnagedcom.com

- **DNA Painter**
  https://dnapainter.com

- **The Leeds Method**
  https://www.danaleeds.com and
  https://genesis.gedmatch.com

- **GEDmatch and GEDmatch Genesis**
  https://www.gedmatch.com and
  https://genesis.gedmatch.com

- **David Pikes' DNA Apps**
  https://www.math.mun.ca/~dapike/FF23utils

Glossary of Terms

Autosomal DNA Segment Analyzer (ADSA): A tool that creates a table for each chromosome with information on each segment though color-coded graphics. Instead of getting a table of numbers, you get a table of colors making it visually easier to find the segments for triangulation.

Automatic clustering: The process of using an automated computer program to sort through your DNA matches from a DNA testing company for you and group them into family groups for you. The groups are displayed in a colorful chart or grid, with each color typically reflecting people related to you by DNA through a certain biological grandparent or grandparents.

Autosomal DNA: The genetic material located in the nucleus of the cell which consists of chromosomes 1-22.

Brick wall: A dead end in genealogy research on a line of ancestors or branch in the family tree. Reasons for this are varied, such as family records stop, you lack access to records to ancestors who lived or were born in a different country, records were lost due to a fire or flood, and many others.

Carrier screening (including expanded carrier screening): Medical DNA testing that looks for recessive gene variants that a person is unaware is being passed down through the family, as carriers of them have no symptoms or illness from it. Today, it is more common for everyone to receive a screen of many conditions before or during their childbearing years. These large tests have been called pan-ethnic, universal, or expanded carrier screening.

Centimorgan (cM): A unit used solely in the measurement of DNA and is a relative distance along the length of a chromosome rather than an actual physical difference.

Chromosome: A DNA-and-protein structure in the nucleus of a cell that contains genetic information. There are 23 matched pairs of chromosomes in most humans (two copies of chromosome 1, two copies of chromosomes 2, etc.). There are some variations from exact pairing (e.g. most individuals with Down syndrome have three full copies of chromosome 21 rather than two).

Chromosome browser: A specific tool available from a DNA testing company or independent site that allows you to see where there is shared DNA between two or more individuals in that company or independent site's database.

Confidential Intermediary (CI): A person who can be involved in managing the release of information to and communication between an adoptee and birth relatives. Certified CIs are individuals with special training and certification regarding records access for adoptees and birth parents.

Diagnostic testing: One category of DNA testing that a doctor might order. "Diagnostic" means the test is used to look for a root cause in a person's DNA, to clarify the reason for that person's condition, illness, or disease.

DNAGedcom: A website created by genetic genealogists who were helping adoptees search for birth parents. This site allows users who have tested at multiple companies to upload their data into one place and begin further analysis.

Ethnicity: The state of belonging to a group of individuals because of a common national or cultural tradition.

Exome test: One of the most extensive versions of medical DNA testing currently available, typically only focusing on the 1-2% of our DNA that is composed of genes.

Expanded carrier screen: A sub-type of carrier screening that analyzes the risk for multiple disorders with a single sample without taking into consideration the tester's ethnic background.

Foundling: An individual who was found abandoned by its parent(s) as an infant or child, discovered, and then cared for by others.

Fully identical region (FIR): Segments of DNA where two people match on both the inherited maternal and paternal chromosomes.

Genealogical cousin: A cousin who is a relative based on genealogy research and placed on someone's family tree because of records (not DNA).

Genealogical tree: A chart derived from record research concerning a person's ancestry.

Genetic counselor: A professional with masters-level training in medical genetics and counseling. They advise people on risks, support informed decision-making around testing, and help interpret the results of DNA testing.

Genetic cousin: A cousin who is a DNA match to the tester because they have descended from a common ancestor.

Genetic genealogist: Individuals who have become adept at using DNA information to piece together how individuals and their families are connected. They may use information from DNA testing combined with genealogical research to construct a person's possible family tree.

Genetic sexual attraction (GSA): A term that describes the unexpected feeling of romantic attraction between biological relatives and has been known to occur in some situations of family members meeting for the first time as adults.

Genetic tree: A chart consisting of DNA matches showing the descent from a common ancestor or ancestors.

Genome test: One of the most extensive versions of testing currently available which tests almost all of a person's DNA. Some people use the term "whole genome test" interchangeably, although referring to the test this way can be misleading.

Genome-wide association study (GWAS): A study of a large group of people that looks for "hotspots" in the genome that might be associated with diseases or traits, requiring different follow-up studies to confirm and understand the association.

Genetic Information Non-discrimination Act (GINA) of 2008: A United States federal law that protects individuals from genetic discrimination in some situations involving health insurance and employment. Genetic discrimination is the misuse of genetic information to make unfair decisions that infringe on a person's rights (to apply and receive insurance, be hired or fired, etc.). GNA is Canada's similar law.

Half-identical region (HIR): Areas of a chromosome where one segment of DNA on either the maternal or paternal chromosome exactly matches another person.

Haplogroup: A genetic population group of people who share a common ancestor on their direct maternal or paternal line.

Heteroplasmy: The state of having more than one type of mitochondrial DNA pattern in one person's cells. It is both common and normal but can create unclear test results.

Identical by Descent (IBD): When two or more people share an identical segment of DNA from a common ancestor without any change to that DNA segment.

Identical by State (IBS): When two people have matching segments, but it is by chance rather than due to the individuals sharing a common ancestor. This situation leads to many false positive results in databases when you are only looking at very small segments of DNA (1-5+ cM values).

Identifying information (ID): Information in some birth and adoption records that can identify individual people and distinguish them from others in the population. This is used in contrast to non-identifying (non-ID) information. Examples are the actual first and last name of a birth mother or father.

JWorks: An Excel-based tool combines the results from the major testing companies for streamlined analysis.

Kworks: A tool that runs on your browser and will sort and group results from chromosome browsers.

Leeds method: A method of sorting matches into family groups, each assigned different colors to allow the user to look for patterns that help solve the family search.

Match: A person who shares identifiable DNA segments with you because you have an ancestor or ancestors in common. The more DNA you share with a match, the more closely related you are to them.

Matrix tool: A tool that helps determine if potential triangulation groups fall on a person's maternal or paternal side.

Microchimerism: A condition where there are cells within the body representing more than one DNA profile. It can happen naturally or as a result of a medical procedure (such as a bone marrow or stem cell transplant). Quality control issues with a raw data file can sometimes be falsely mistaken as evidence of microchimerism.

Mirror trees: A technique to help identify an unknown common ancestor by duplicating the genealogy tree of a match and attaching your DNA result to it to determine which descendants you match, and from which line(s), in their tree.

Mitochondria: An energy-producing organelle found in large numbers within a person's cell and frequently described as the "powerhouse" of the cell.

Mitochondrial DNA: The genetic material inside of mitochondria shaped into a 16,500 base pair ring allowing researchers to trace their direct maternal line.

MRCA (most recent common ancestor): The most recent individual or couple from whom two or more people are directly descended, commonly a grandparent or great-grandparent couple for 1st or 2nd cousins.

Non-identifying information (non-ID): Some birth and adoption documents contain information about individuals that is general and cannot be used to distinguish them from others in the population. This is used in contrast to identifying (ID) information. Examples are the age or general health history of a birth mother or father.

Not the Parent Expected (NPE): The term for people who make the discovery that their parent(s) are not biologically related to them, previously known as a non-paternal event and also currently referred to as misattributed parentage.

Pharmacogenomic testing (PGx): A type of specialized DNA testing that looks at certain DNA variants in genes that influence an individual's reactions to certain medications.

Phasing: The process of determining which parent (mother or father) contributed which DNA letter to their child at a specific location in the DNA.

Placebo-controlled study: A type of study which pits placebo pills or treatment given to one group of people against a pill or treatment with active ingredients to see if the active ingredients have any effect.

Polygenic: A term that refers to a condition or trait that is determined by a large number of genes rather than just one or a few. Many common conditions are polygenic (most forms of diabetes, heart disease, lupus, etc.).

Proactive screening: A type of medical DNA testing that allows people to gain more information about their potential medical risks but without risking more. Also known as preventative screening.

Raw data: The .vcf (or sometimes .csv or .xml) file a tester can download from a testing company which contains the DNA data from the sample which was submitted. Other types of raw data files exist for use in bioinformatics but are not the kind used for genealogical research purposes.

Reference population: A selection of people representing groups from around the world whose DNA markers are used by testing companies. The entire set of data from a group of people is called the reference data set, and the people in it are referred to as the reference population.

Registry: A set of information (usually name and contact information) used for any different number of reasons.

Run of Homozygosity (ROH): A stretch of DNA markers that are identical for that region inherited from the mother and also from the father. ROH is a common DNA feature for all people, and it is seen in higher-than-average levels in people who have endogamy in their family or whose parents are close relatives.

Segment: A chunk of DNA on a chromosome determined by a start location and an end location on the chromosome.

Search angel: An experienced researcher who volunteers their time to individual cases typically because they have been through a search for biological family themselves or on behalf of someone they know, and they want to share their skills to help others.

Visual phasing: A specific type of phasing that focuses on the appearance of matching regions between DNA relatives, typically using a chromosome browser.

Vital record: Any record kept under government authority such as birth certificate, marriage license, or death certificate that officially documents a major life event.

Variants of Uncertain Significance (VUS): A DNA letter change in a gene that might be cause for disease or might have no effect on our bodies, for which further information is needed in order to know.

X chromosome: A human sex chromosome, two of which are typically present in genetic female cells (shown as XX) and one in male cells (shown as XY).

Y chromosome: A human sex chromosome, typically present only in genetic male cells, shown as XY.

Author Biographies

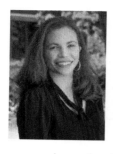

Brianne Kirkpatrick, MS, LCGC is a licensed and certified genetic counselor with a medical genetics background who now specializes in the area of ancestry testing. She is the founder of Watershed DNA and works with clients who are impacted by adoption, donor conception, and NPE (not the parent expected) discoveries. Brianne first used genetic genealogy for her own family research and writes and blogs to help others understand the various types of genetic testing. She is passionate about helping others to understand DNA and encourages clear and compassionate communication around sensitive family topics.

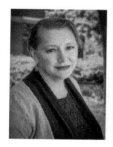

Shannon Combs-Bennett, QG, PLCGS is an author and lecturer within the genealogical community. She writes and speaks nationally and internationally on a variety of traditional genealogy topics and genetic genealogy. Shannon is the founder and owner of Trials and Tribulations (T2) Family History where she works with clients to solve their genealogical, and genetic, questions. She earned her BS in biology and is currently earning her MSc in Genealogic, Heraldic, and Paleographic Studies. Shannon's book *Genealogy Basics in 30 Minutes* won the IBPA Benjamin Franklin Silver Award and the Mother's Choice Award for hobby books in 2017.

Disclosures: The authors are not affiliated with and do not receive compensation from any of the DNA testing companies or third party sites/tools mentioned or not mentioned this book. Brianne is a volunteer on the advisory board to the MyHeritage "DNA Quest" program for kit donations for use by adoptees/birth family.

Acknowledgements

We authors would like to recognize our families for the unwavering support during the process of creating this book. To Michael, Owen, Emily, and Henry, and to Kelly, Kieran, and Euan: thank you for your love and patience as we threw our hearts and time into this project!

We would also like to acknowledge the participants in the genetic genealogy community, some but unfortunately not all of whom received specific mention in the chapters and/or resources. There are so many that listing individually by name would be an additional chapter.

Finally, we would not have been able to put together all this information and advice without adoptees in the online genealogy community, our clients, family, and others we have spoken with in person. The interactions we have had over the past few years with the many people affected by an adoption (of themselves or a family member's) have made the greatest impact on this book. Your stories were the inspiration for every part, chapter, and bullet point.

Index

Human Genome Project, 159

Huntington's disease, 166, 174

Hutterite, 151

Identical By Descent, 104-105

Identical By State, 104

incest, 34

Institute for Genetic Genealogy, 65

international adoption, 22, 23

International Society for Genetic Genealogy, 97, 108, 110-111, 118-119, 134

Kirkpatrick, Brianne, 11-12, 17, 47, 79, 133, 147, 183, 191, 194, 223

Kits of Kindness, 118

late-discovery adoptees, 46

law enforcement, 141

Legacy Family Tree Webinars, 65

legal rights, 20-21

legislation, 20, 53, 197

life insurance, 161, 190

living people, 42

macular degeneration, 179

maternal relatives, 46

medical conditions, 15, 67, 77

medical DNA tests, 77, 161

medical history, 13, 19, 68, 77-78, 144-145, 161-163, 165, 167-168, 193-194, 199

medical information, 87, 157, 175, 184, 195, 201

megabase pairs, 129

Mendel, Gegor, 95

metabolic disorders, 186

microchimerism, 110

Microsoft Excel, 127

minor children, 9, 197

mitochondria, 96, 110, 111

most recent common ancestor, 130

motivating factors, 13

MRCA. *See* most common recent ancestor

National Genealogical Society, 64

National Society of Genetic Counselors, 199

neurologic disorders, 174

newspapers.com, 102

not the parent expected, 91

nutrigenomics, 186

nutrition, 184

nutritional supplements, 186

online support groups, 46, 85

oral history, 92

outcome
  acceptance, 12

52517565R00133

Made in the USA
Middletown, DE
10 July 2019